# IMPROVING
## NURSE RETENTION
### &
# HEALTHCARE
# OUTCOMES

*Innovating With the **IMPACT** Model*

Judy Thomas, MSN, RN, NEA-BC
Mellisa Renter, MSN, RN, CPN

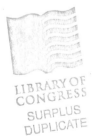

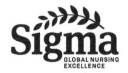

Sigma
GLOBAL NURSING
EXCELLENCE

*Sigma Theta Tau International Honor Society of Nursing (Sigma) is a nonprofit organization whose mission is developing nurse leaders anywhere to improve healthcare everywhere. Founded in 1922, Sigma has more than 135,000 active members in over 100 countries and territories. Members include practicing nurses, instructors, researchers, policymakers, entrepreneurs, and others. Sigma's more than 540 chapters are located at more than 700 institutions of higher education throughout Armenia, Australia, Botswana, Brazil, Canada, Colombia, England, Eswatini, Ghana, Hong Kong, Ireland, Israel, Jamaica, Japan, Jordan, Kenya, Lebanon, Malawi, Mexico, the Netherlands, Nigeria, Pakistan, Philippines, Portugal, Puerto Rico, Scotland, Singapore, South Africa, South Korea, Sweden, Taiwan, Tanzania, Thailand, the United States, and Wales. Learn more at www.sigmanursing.org.*

**Sigma Theta Tau International | 550 West North Street, Indianapolis, IN, USA 46202**

To request a review copy for course adoption, order additional books, buy in bulk, or purchase for corporate use, contact Sigma Marketplace at 888.654.4968 (US/Canada toll-free), +1.317.687.2256 (International), or solutions@sigmamarketplace.org.

To request author information, or for speaker or other media requests, contact Sigma Marketing at 888.634.7575 (US/Canada toll-free) or +1.317.634.8171 (International).

ISBN: 9781646480463 | EPUB ISBN: 9781646480470 | PDF ISBN: 9781646480487 | MOBI ISBN: 9781646480494

Library of Congress Cataloging-in-Publication Data
Names: Thomas, Judy, 1969- author. | Renter, Mellisa, 1986- author.

Title: Improving nurse retention & healthcare outcomes : innovating with the IMPACT model / Judy Thomas, Mellisa Renter.

Other titles: Improving nurse retention and healthcare outcomes

Description: Indianapolis, IN : Sigma Theta Tau International Honor Society of Nursing [2021] | Includes bibliographical references and index. | Summary: "Nurse retention is a key focus for healthcare organizations-particularly the retention of clinical nurses, who provide direct patient care. The costs associated with nurse turnover can have a huge impact on a hospital's profit margin. Additionally, nurse turnover affects job satisfaction among clinical nurses, which leads to burnout, making it even harder to provide safe care to patients and to achieve overall organizational initiatives. Bottom line: Nurse turnover has a multidimensional effect on an organization's ability to thrive. Considering the various reasons clinical nurses leave the direct patient care role, authors Judy Thomas and Melissa Renter created the IMPACT Program to stimulate empowerment and professional growth, which lead to increased job satisfaction-ultimately improving retention and helping nurses thrive in their roles"— Provided by publisher.

Identifiers: LCCN 2021014162 (print) | LCCN 2021014163 (ebook) | ISBN 9781646480463 (paperback) | ISBN 9781646480470 (epub) | ISBN 9781646480487 (adobe pdf) | ISBN 9781646480494 (kindle edition)
Subjects: MESH: Nursing—organization & administration | Nurses—psychology | Personnel Management—methods | Quality of Health Care—standards Classification: LCC RT89 (print) | LCC RT89 (ebook) | NLM WY 30 | DDC 362.17/3068—dc23
LC record available at https://lccn.loc.gov/2021014162
LC ebook record available at https://lccn.loc.gov/2021014163

First Printing, 2021

**Publisher:** Dustin Sullivan

**Acquisitions Editor:** Emily Hatch

**Development Editor:** Kate Shoup

**Cover Designer:** TNT Design Inc.

**Interior Design/Page Layout:** Michael Tanamachi

**Indexer:** Larry Sweazy

**Managing Editor:** Carla Hall

**Publications Specialist:** Todd Lothery

**Project Editor:** Kate Shoup

**Copy Editor:** Todd Lothery

**Proofreader:** Gill Editorial Services

# FREE BOOK RESOURCES

You can download a sample chapter and forms for this book from the Sigma Repository. Visit this book's page by following the link or taking a smartphone photo of the QR code below.

http://hdl.handle.net/10755/21457

# DEDICATION

Judy dedicates this book to her amazing husband, Scott, for his constant support and for always being there for each new adventure she takes, like writing this book. She also dedicates this book to her wonderful children, Eryn and Evan, who have made her proud in every way.

Mellisa dedicates this book to her superhuman husband, Jake, who held down the fort while she checked off this bucket-list item, and to her two children, Riley and Charlotte, who are her inspiration and reminder that these are the good old days. Always make the most of your day, little ones. Team Renter!

# ACKNOWLEDGMENTS

We would like to thank the executive leadership of Children's Hospital & Medical Center. Your dedication to transformational leadership has motivated and inspired us to create amazing initiatives and programs within the organization. We would also like to thank the nursing leadership team. Your commitment to engaging in the professional growth of our staff is unwavering and greatly appreciated. Lastly, we would like to thank our incredible clinical nurses, who are the foundation of our organization. Your innovation and creativity are awe-inspiring. Thank you for your intentional focus and commitment to provide the highest quality of care.

# ABOUT THE AUTHORS

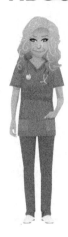

**Judy Thomas, MSN, RN, NEA-BC**, is the Service Line Director for the Hematology/Oncology & Infusion Center at Children's Hospital & Medical Center in Omaha, Nebraska. Previously, she held the position of Director of Professional Nursing Practice and Magnet® Program Director at Children's. Before joining Children's in 2015, she was the Pediatric Manager at the Nebraska Medical Center. In 2017, she received the Nursing Leadership Award and a DAISY Award.

Thomas's academic career began as a BSN graduate in nursing. She then earned a master's degree in nursing leadership, for which she was awarded the Academic Excellence Award. During the course of her 25-year career, Thomas has served as a certified nursing assistant, a hospital-based RN, a home healthcare RN, a charge nurse, a manager, a director, and a nursing instructor.

Thomas is Nurse Executive Advanced Board Certified (NEA-BC), a PROSI Certified Change Management Practitioner, a Fundamentals of Magnet certificate holder; and a trained Language of Caring educator. With her Gallup strengths of Relator, Developer, Strategic, Restorative, and Woo, she has a talent for leading teams through the journeys of engagement, retention, and recruitment and toward positive outcomes.

You will *never* find Thomas eating anything that swims or a vegetable, as she truly prefers the kids' menu at any restaurant.

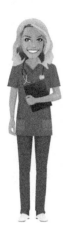

**Mellisa Renter, MSN, RN, CPN**, is the Director of Professional Nursing Practice and Magnet® Program Director at Children's Hospital & Medical Center in Omaha, Nebraska. Previously, she served as a Clinical Education Specialist for the ambulatory specialty clinics at Children's.

Renter graduated with a bachelor of science in nursing in 2008 and with a master's of science in nursing education in 2013. During her 12-year nursing career, Renter has held various roles in the ambulatory care setting as a direct patient care nurse. She has also worked in academia, teaching bachelor's-prepared nursing students. Most recently she served as a member of nursing leadership.

Renter is the recipient of the 2019 March of Dimes Nurse of the Year Award in Pediatric Excellence. She is a PROSCI Certified Change Management Practitioner. In 2014 her article "How Magnet® Designation Affects Nurse Retention: An Evidence-Based Research Project" was published in the *American Nurse Today* journal.

Renter's Gallup strengths of Futuristic, Discipline, Focus, Learner, and Significance have all guided her to success. Her passion to empower and engage nurses through professional development, create healthy work environments to thrive, and establish cross-continuum connectedness have been foundational elements of her career path.

In her spare time, you will find Renter wearing a baseball cap and leggings, cheering on her beautiful children from the sidelines in one of their multiple sports year-round, or shopping at Target.

# TABLE OF CONTENTS

# FOREWORD

As Chief Nursing Officer at Children's Hospital & Medical Center in Omaha, Nebraska, for nearly 30 years, I have spent much of my career working to unlock the secret to retaining excellent direct clinical care nurses. Today, more than ever, nurses have many career choices. Establishing a career identity, often defined as upward mobility, can pull them away from direct patient care. Clinical care nursing is hard work, and this, too, can lead nurses to pursue other paths.

At Children's, we have searched for ways to create a long-term career path for clinical care nurses that is attractive and rewarding. Along the way, we tried various traditional "fixes": career ladders, special shifts, incentive pay, and more. However, none of these methods led to lasting or meaningful improvement.

Two motivated nurse leaders, Mellisa Renter and Judy Thomas, were undaunted by this challenge, fueled by their belief in the extraordinary impact of the clinical nurse and a passion for nursing excellence. They set out to develop an innovative model that would make a positive difference in retaining clinical nurses, complete with practical, effective techniques that address the needs of not only the nurse but also patient outcomes and the organization. In the process, they emerged as true thought leaders and systems thinkers; their work impressed audiences in the boardroom and the patient room.

As we measured and attained positive outcomes within the organization and shared the program with others via national and local podium presentations, outside organizational leaders reached out seeking information on steps to implement the program within their own systems. They were in need of some proven keys to unlock a meaningful solution. Out of this need and a desire to support direct clinical nurses everywhere, Renter and Thomas wrote *Improving Nurse Retention & Healthcare Outcomes: Innovating With the IMPACT Model*. This book provides the theory behind the model, real-life techniques, and a step-by-step implementation guide. The beauty of this approach is that it elevates nursing practice through the use of evidenced-based practice, research, and performance improvement, with outcomes associated. This program has been a game changer for our organization, and I know it will be for yours, as well.

— **Kathy English**, MSN, MBA, RN, NE-BC, FACHE
Executive Vice President,
Chief Operating Officer, & Chief Nursing Officer
Executive Administration
Children's Hospital & Medical Center, Omaha, Nebraska

# INTRODUCTION

*"Are we prepared to leave our comfort zones to reach a better place?"*

–Elder Carlos A. Godoy

In 2015, we joined Children's Hospital & Medical Center (Children's) in Omaha, Nebraska. Within months, our paths crossed when we were asked to colead an initiative to improve nurse retention. Together, we led a team in the creation and implementation of a new and innovative recognition and reward model. This program not only improved the organization's direct patient care nurse retention rate but also had a profound impact on the professionalism of our nursing staff and on various organizational strategic initiatives.

Nurse retention is a key focus for healthcare organizations—particularly the retention of clinical nurses, who provide direct patient care. The costs associated with nurse turnover can have a huge impact on a hospital's profit margin. In fact, each percent change in nurse turnover (or retention) will cost (or save) the average hospital an additional $306,400 per year. Moreover, the cost of turnover per nurse ranges from $33,300 to $56,000 (NSI Nursing Solutions, 2020). This turnover then leads to hospitals losing on average $5.2 million to $8.0 million annually due to bedside nurse turnover (Vaughn, 2020).

Nurse turnover in a hospital setting doesn't just have financial implications. It also has a direct impact on the remaining clinical nurses themselves, which then trickles down to patient care. For example, when a nurse leaves an organization, it often becomes challenging to ensure safe staffing standards and the right skill mix to provide high-quality care. This in turn affects job satisfaction among clinical nurses, which may lead to burnout, making it even harder to provide safe care to patients and to achieve overall organizational initiatives. Bottom line: Nurse turnover has a multidimensional effect on an organization's ability to thrive.

One of the biggest mistakes an organization can make is to react to turnover of clinical nurses as it occurs rather than develop a sustainable retention process for these critical staff members. We call this the "Band-Aid" approach. It's a quick fix with limited benefits. At Children's, our nursing leadership team understood that we needed to look beyond short-term fixes and take a more proactive and sustainable approach toward retention.

To achieve this, we wanted to create a model to motivate nurses to remain as frontline staff. We envisioned a proactive program that would enable us to empower nurses, engage them, and ultimately retain them. We had long observed that empowerment and engagement were closely linked—and that a lack of empowerment created a lack of engagement. This in turn caused a vicious cycle that ultimately led clinical nurses to leave the organization or the nursing profession altogether (see Figure I.1).

## LACK OF EMPOWERMENT EFFECT

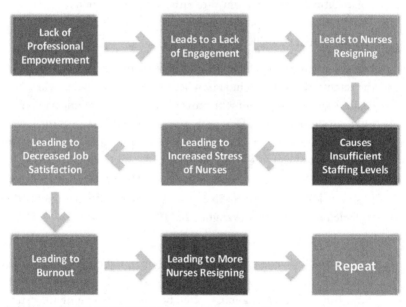

**FIGURE I.1** Effect on nurse retention and a lack of empowerment.

This program would be very different from past initiatives, as it would intentionally focus on the more upstream causes of this vicious cycle rather than downstream effects. We also saw an opportunity to leverage empowerment and engagement to influence other aspects of the organization, such as our strategic initiatives, mission, and vision.

We wanted to think innovatively to positively influence nurse retention. It was time to dream of *all* the possibilities. We asked ourselves:

- What if we could ignite nursing professional growth to drive retention?

- What if we could ingrain a culture of empowerment and engagement to help influence our organization's strategic initiatives, mission, and vision?

- What if we could address the needs of our patients and positively influence outcomes across the continuum of care?

These *what-ifs* were the driving forces to think differently about typical retention initiatives.

Then we considered the various reasons clinical nurses leave the direct patient care role. Some do it to pursue further education—which is greatly needed and which we completely support. Some do it to assume a leadership role. Again, that's great. But a great many clinical nurses don't necessarily *want* to leave the direct patient care role; they simply feel they have to if they want to grow professionally.

This observation really struck the Children's leadership team. We realized that we just didn't offer many avenues for professional advancement for clinical nurses. So, we set forth to create one. We called it the IMPACT Model.

We designed the IMPACT Model, or Program, to stimulate empowerment and professional growth. We believed this would lead to increased job satisfaction—which would in turn improve retention. Simply put, we wanted our clinical nurses to thrive in their role. We wanted them to know that they had not only made a difference in their day-to-day shift but also had an effect on the future care of patients they serve. That's what the IMPACT Model is all about.

This book outlines what the IMPACT Model is, how it works, and what it has achieved. No matter your role—whether you are an executive or a clinical nurse—this book will resonate with you. If you are a clinical nurse, you will gain a clear understanding of how you can elevate your practice as a frontline direct patient care provider. You will be inspired to create change—not only in your unit or area but across your organization. Your job will no longer be about simply clocking in, doing your shift, and clocking back out. It will be about being empowered to improve patient care and your work environment and helping lead your organization into the future of healthcare. If you are an executive/leader, this book will open your eyes to a new way of approaching clinical nurse retention that will also positively influence your strategic initiatives. You will gain a new perspective on becoming a more transformational leader, enabling those closest to the work to lead your organization to meet its strategic goals.

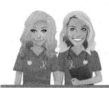 **GOOD IDEA**

This book focuses primarily on clinical nurse retention. But with a few tweaks, the IMPACT Model can be used to improve retention for any role within your organization that affects your organization's mission, vision, and strategic initiatives—for example, physical therapy, occupational therapy, pharmacy, nurse practitioner, clinical nurse specialist, educator, respiratory therapy, and so on. Remember: Retention is essential for all roles.

We can't wait to share our innovative approach to nurse retention with you! Before we begin, though, here's a quick rundown:

- Chapter 1 outlines the retention practices commonly used by most organizations. As you'll see, these practices are often nothing more than short-term fixes. They only see you through the immediate crisis, are quite costly, and offer little return on investment in terms of overall strategic initiatives.

- Chapter 2 discusses the key stakeholders and instrumental decision points in the creation of our program to improve nurse retention.

- Chapter 3 takes a high-level look at the structure of the IMPACT Model.

- Chapters 4–7 offer step-by-step details on each phase of the IMPACT Model.

- Chapter 8 describes the type of leadership commitment it takes to start and sustain a program of this magnitude.

- Chapter 9 explains how we obtained leadership buy-in from the get-go to begin the process of developing a program and achieved broader organizational buy-in to sustain it once it was off the ground.

- Chapter 10 reveals outcomes from specific IMPACT Model projects completed by participating nurses as well as broader organizational gains associated with the IMPACT Model.

- Chapter 11 showcases the professional journey of clinical nurses as they navigate the program. You will gain a greater perspective on how the IMPACT Model empowers clinical nurses, who spend the majority of their time on the front lines.

We are confident that you will see how implementing an initiative like the IMPACT Model will not only improve your clinical nurse retention rate but also influence your ability to tackle strategic initiatives within your organization. We can't wait to guide you on your journey!

# *REFERENCES*

NSI Nursing Solutions. (2020). *2020 NSI national health care retention & RN staffing report*. https://www.nsinursingsolutions.com/Documents/Library/NSI_National_Health_Care_Retention_Report.pdf

Vaughn, N. (2020, October 27). *Nurse turnover rates: How to reduce healthcare turnover*. https://www.relias.com/blog/how-to-reduce-healthcare-turnover

*"If you can dream it, you can do it."*

—Walt Disney

## CHAPTER 1

# Traditional Nurse Retention Practices

## INTRODUCTION

For many nurse leaders, the topic of retention rarely creeps into our conversations. Instead, it comes barreling in when we hit crisis mode. When this happens, we slowly dig ourselves out—and then, BAM! We are right in it again. This is crazy!

Simply put, we are reactionary. Rather than planning ahead to prevent problems like staff shortages, we react to them when they occur. We seek a quick fix, doing whatever we believe will get us through the moment. Often, this amounts to offering incentives—say, extra pay (above and beyond overtime) for picking up extra shifts. Then, when the problem is resolved, we revoke these incentives. This inevitably upsets the staff, causing some to refuse to pick up extra shifts because they no longer receive extra pay or to quit altogether. And so, you find yourself short-staffed again, and the whole cycle of giving and taking away begins anew. With the national nursing turnover rate already ranging from 8.8% to 37%, and an aging workforce where approximately 1 million nurses (one-third of the workforce) will reach retirement within the next 10 to 15 years, being reactionary is no longer the answer (Haddad et al. 2020).

In our experience, this reactionary approach of offering incentives during a time of need and then revoking them when things are back to "normal" just creates more headaches for us as leaders. It's always an up-hill battle, and it's exhausting. It's far better to develop a long-term plan for retaining nurses—one that incorporates several different approaches.

This chapter outlines just a few traditional practices for nurse retention (and recruitment). As you'll see, although these practices sometimes have their place, they don't do much to solve the long-term issue of nurse retention.

## JUDY

Back in my day—which was admittedly quite some time ago—nurses were told when we were expected to arrive for our shifts and when we were expected to leave, and that was about all. We just did our jobs, no questions asked. Well, times have changed, and we need to change with them. We must take a hard look at what we do and ask ourselves, is it working? Is it a long-term solution? On a related note, we must process the needs and wants of members of various generations in terms of feeling fulfilled in the workplace. Giving temporary incentives is like placing a Band-Aid on a wound. Eventually, you have to rip it off—and it is painful!

# CURRENT RETENTION PRACTICES

There are many common practices to retain and even recruit clinical nurses. These practices apply when we are navigating short-term staffing crises as well as when the development of new programs requires increased staffing numbers. Historically, the most common of these have included the following:

- Hire-on bonus

- Tuition reimbursement

- Shift bonuses

- Seniority considerations
- Career ladders

## *Hire-On Bonus*

A *hire-on bonus* is given to new hires to incentivize them to remain employed for a set period of time. It achieves this by delaying payment of the full bonus until said period of time has passed.

Offering hire-on bonuses might enable you to attract some amazing nurses who actually stay past the payout period. But let's be real: You'll also attract nurses who just want the bonus—and will bolt the minute they get it.

Additionally, the financial impact is quite high—and not in a good way with respect to long-term return on investment. A hire-on bonus payout can range from $1,000 to $10,000 on average (Uzuegbunem, n.d.). Some bonuses have been known to go as high as $40,000 if it is a "hard to fill role." A typical hire-on bonus requires a clinical nurse to stay approximately three years, with no real commitment to the organization beyond fulfilling their shift requirements. So, although this financial incentive temporarily fixes one problem (staffing), it does not help the organization meet any of its larger strategic initiatives. All you accomplish is paying more to fulfill a staffing need. And, when the three years is up, you are likely right back where you started: out one clinical nurse—who, by the way, now has more experience and is therefore even more valuable than before.

Finally, and most importantly (in our opinion), is the effect of hire-on bonuses on current staff, some of whom may have devoted many years to your organization. Often, hire-on bonuses cause current staff to feel undervalued, especially if they received no such bonus when they were hired. Hire-on bonuses may also create animosity between current staff and new hires. So, not only do hire-on bonuses offer only a temporary fix to staffing issues, they also may result in job dissatisfaction for your experienced nurses.

## Tuition Reimbursement

Like hire-on bonuses, offering tuition reimbursement is a recruitment tactic that ideally results in improved retention. But as with hire-on bonuses, offering tuition reimbursement can cause multiple problems for your organization:

- Offering tuition reimbursement is expensive and may not be sustainable.

- There's nothing to stop nurses from working just as long as is needed to pay off their loans before departing for a job elsewhere.

- It offers little value beyond the obvious extra pair of hands for a select number of years.

- Current staff who were not offered tuition reimbursement may grow resentful.

## Shift Bonuses

All too often, when organizations reach high census or high vacancy levels and need nurse coverage stat, they offer shift bonuses—extra money in addition to overtime—on a temporary basis. While it's true that offering shift bonuses can help in the short term, this practice often creates new problems down the line. If you as a nurse leader have ever asked someone to pick up a shift or perform some other above-and-beyond task, only to be asked, "Are you offering a bonus for that?" you know what we're talking about!

## Seniority Considerations

Many organizations reward long-term employees by moving them from night or weekend shifts to more "regular" hours. But this practice creates a whole new set of problems—for those with tenure and those without. For example:

- Are these moves guaranteed after a certain period of time?

- What if staffing changes require more senior nurses to move back to nights or weekends?

- How do these moves affect their peers?
- If you have good retention rates, will new hires *ever* get nights or weekends off?

## Career Ladders

Career ladders have been used for years as a promotional progression structure for employees. The purpose of this structure is typically thought of in two ways:

- **To enable employees to take advantage of educational opportunities to advance in their career:** For example, in the healthcare industry, an organization might recruit certified nursing assistants in entry-level roles—the bottom rung on the career ladder. If these nursing assistants want to move up the ladder, the organization supports them as they attend school to become nurses. If these employees continue to advance educationally—for example, to take on roles such as nurse practitioner, clinical nurse specialist, nurse educator, nurse manager, and so on—the career ladder structure supports them in their journey and increases their salary accordingly.

- **As a professional tool for growth:** As nurses gain experience and expertise, they can move up the career ladder to a higher level and higher paying positions.

As you can see, career ladders serve the purpose of encouraging staff to move their career away from practicing at the bedside into higher roles with more responsibility, authority, and higher pay (Health eCareers, 2010). Now, it is great that we retain and look to help our nursing workforce in advancing their career, but not all nurses seek this or want it, and they may feel then like they have few growth avenues in their role as a clinical nurse. The career ladder approach also does not focus on aligning the growth of the clinical nurse toward meeting overall strategic organizational initiatives; it is truly just focused on individual nurses and their future career.

# TIME TO THINK DIFFERENTLY

Offering hire-on bonuses, tuition reimbursement, and shift bonuses, considering seniority, and supporting a career ladder have their place. But most are just temporary practices to get you through difficult times. Moreover, some are quite costly, with little to no return on investment in terms of meeting the organization's overall strategic initiatives. Still, we often find ourselves with no choice but to institute these practices from time to time to react to particular staffing challenges.

It is time to think differently—to look toward a long-term, sustainable solution to meet overall organizational initiatives. We need to ask ourselves two important questions:

- Why are our clinical nurses leaving the front line?
- Is there a way to motivate them to stay and drive the future of patient care?

Too often, experienced nurses move away from the direct care of patients. Some do so to advance their education—and rightfully so. Others, however, are simply searching for opportunities for professional growth and fulfillment—opportunities that don't seem to exist at the front line. As nurses continue to leave their direct care roles for these reasons, a third reason begins to arise: emotional constrain with being short-staffed (Buchan & Aiken, 2008). So, they leave the front line to pursue other opportunities, continuing the vicious cycle of low staffing and the need to institute the practices discussed in this chapter.

This needs fixing. Simply put, we need to change the clinical nurse role to make it more of a career and not just a job. That's what this book is about.

# CREATING A CAREER AT THE BEDSIDE

What's the difference between a *job* and a career? A job is often a short-term work commitment—you join the workforce to earn a paycheck. There's rarely any passion involved, nor is there a desire or commitment to stay long term. In contrast, a *career* is work that provides opportunities for professional and personal growth. People with a career feel supported and compensated for their contributions, which ultimately leads to a long-term commitment.

Our organization, Children's Hospital & Medical Center, in Omaha, Nebraska, wanted clinical nurses to be able to make a long-term commitment to remain on the front lines, or bedside, to care for patients—in other words, to pursue a career at the bedside. To achieve this, we needed a better understanding of what drives clinical nursing staff to stay on the front lines to care for those who need them the most. We began by identifying non-negotiable must-haves for both clinical nurses and the organization as a whole to serve as guiding principles. These were as follows:

- Clinical nurse retention

- Increased clinical nurse job enjoyment

- Increased clinical nurse autonomy, professional development, and advocacy

- Interprofessional collaboration

- Forward movement of the organization's mission, vision, and strategic initiatives

- Improved organizational outcomes

- Improved patient outcomes

- Increased evidenced-based, research, and performance improvement projects

- Cross-continuum alignment

- Financial stewardship

- Connection to national designations

At first we tried to create the traditional career ladder to account for each of these guiding principles. But we soon found out this was impossible. So, we decided to create something different and broader from scratch: a model that focused on clinical nurse professional advancement in a whole new way. Working with a team of leaders and staff, and using our guiding principles as a road map, we embarked on a journey to create a sustainable solution to promote a career at the bedside.

## JUDY

Early in my career, I knew that leadership was where my heart was. My master's program was focused on transformational leadership and staff engagement. As a past and current leader of multiple areas in a healthcare setting, I was passionate about leading staff. I especially wanted to involve staff in creating solutions for anything we were looking to change that affected them. Advancing into leadership was and still is the best career choice I have made.

I have now spent the last 20-plus years listening to and working with staff on retention efforts. As leaders, we need to be open to what is truly happening in our organizations. We need to stop making assumptions, take a step back, and let our teams lead with us. You will be amazed at what they will accomplish. Needless to say, this opportunity to create a program where we are promoting a career at the bedside was right up my alley!

## MELLISA

As a nurse for the past 10-plus years, professional development has always held a special place in my heart. I thrived when given professional development opportunities to grow as an ambulatory clinical nurse working with patients.

Knowing the effect these opportunities had on me, I wanted to create them for others. So, I transitioned into leadership, where I could influence and create processes and systems to empower clinical nurses through professional development experiences. Having the opportunity to create a program that focused on empowerment and engagement through professional development was very exciting and aligned with my passion.

# *REFERENCES*

Buchan, J., & Aiken, L. (2008). Solving nursing shortages: A common priority. *Journal of Clinical Nursing, 17*(24), 3262–3268. https://www.ncbi.nlm.nih.gov/pmc/articles/PMC2858425/

Haddad, L. M., Annamaraju, P., & Toney-Butler, T. J. (2020). Nursing shortage. *StatPearls Publishing.* https://www.ncbi.nlm.nih.gov/books/NBK493175/

Health eCareers. (2010, Nov. 2). *About career ladders for nursing.* https://www.healthecareers.com/article/career/about-career-ladders-for-nursing#:~:text=Nursing%20is%20a%20very%20flexible,more%20authority%20and%20better%20salaries

Uzuegbunem, T. (n.d.). Nursing bonus: Everything you need to know. *NurseMoneyTalk.com.* https://nursemoneytalk.com/blog/nursing-bonus

## CHAPTER 2

# Model Creation

## INTRODUCTION

As you learned in Chapter 1, our organization took an innovative approach to developing a nurse retention model rather than a career ladder. You may be wondering how we made that decision. After all, most organizations have a career ladder; why wouldn't we replicate what is known to be the traditional approach to retention?

Well, this decision was not made with the snap of a finger. It involved significant discussion, collaboration, and decision-making with key stakeholders. This chapter describes key stakeholders and instrumental decision points, how we partnered with marketing to brand the model, and our implementation strategy.

## GETTING THE RIGHT PEOPLE IN THE ROOM

Involving the right key stakeholders in the program-development process was key. These stakeholders included the following:

- **Clinical nurses:** Including clinical nurses was fundamental to ensuring that the program would be simple to navigate and exciting to participate in from a user standpoint.

They were the target audience, so their contributions were invaluable.

- **Nurse managers and directors:** This group included experts in the operational elements of the program.

- **Our chief nursing officer (CNO):** This person's buy-in and engagement was crucial.

- **Nurse educators and clinical nurse specialists:** These were experts in the details of operations, as well as in communicating and educating the nursing division.

- **Human resources:** This department was critical to hammering out compensation and soliciting executive support, as well as carrying out recruitment and retention initiatives.

This group comprised a governance committee, which focused on professional advancement, nurse retention, and nurse recognition initiatives within the organization. The objective of the committee—which met on a monthly basis for a period of one year in addition to attending an all-day workshop at an offsite location—was to develop a professional advancement structure for clinical nurses to create a career at the bedside and improve clinical nurse retention.

Having the right key stakeholders, including the CNO, to develop a professional advancement structure proved to be fundamental. Each member of the governance committee played an essential role, bringing unique perspectives and expertise to the group.

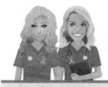

## DREAM TEAM

As the director of professional nursing practice (Judy) and a clinical education specialist (Mellisa), we had the opportunity to serve on the governance committee. In fact, it was while working with this committee that we met and started our professional relationship.

# READY, SET . . . GO!

Once we had assembled the right key stakeholders, the governance committee commenced the journey of developing a professional advancement structure. To begin, we needed to conceptualize a complicated and multifaceted structure that would affect the entire nursing division. (No pressure!)

We decided to start by conducting a literature search to find out what types of structures and programs other healthcare organizations had in place (Children's Hospital & Medical Center [CHMC], 2015). The literature search included a virtual library database and connections with other organizations that were willing to share their structures. This would help us identify the various ways we might approach nurse retention through professional advancement and to pin down best practices.

Our research revealed that many organizations used career ladders to achieve desired professional advancement and retention outcomes. So, the governance committee discussed the pros and cons of career ladders and compared them to our guiding principles and the outcomes we sought. Ultimately, we determined that developing a model that contained the best elements we discovered through our literature search would work better than a career ladder to enable us to reach our goals (CHMC, 2015).

We also felt that developing a program rather than a career ladder would simplify the budgeting processes in relation to base pay and not over-inflating the yearly raise structure (CHMC, 2015). Career ladders typically connect compensation with the various rungs of the ladder. This can get complicated with merit increases, benefits, paid time off, and so on, which can have a huge impact on the organization's budget and bottom line. Utilizing a model approach instead of the career ladder would make it easier to maintain and control the costs associated with it.

This would be a very different approach from other organizations, but we were willing to think outside the box to create something new and innovative!

# LET'S BUILD A MODEL

After we determined that the development of a full program was warranted, committee members worked closely together to hash out the details. To stay focused and to ensure that no foundational elements were overlooked, the committee identified several key decision points, as follows (CHMC, 2015):

- Which clinical nurses would be eligible?
- Would participation be voluntary or involuntary?
- Would there be different levels of achievement?
- What framework would be used to showcase achievement?
- In what activities would participating nurses engage?
- Would the model have objective or subjective measures?
- How would the model connect with the organization's mission, vision, and strategic initiatives?
- How would nurses be compensated for completing the program?
- How would nurses navigate the program autonomously?
- How would nurses demonstrate that they met the model requirements?
- How frequently would the program be offered for participation?

## Eligibility

We set the eligibility criteria as follows (CHMC, 2015):

- **Clinical nurses must work directly with patients at least 50% of the time:** This aligns with national designation standards.
- **Nurses must work at least 20 hours per week:** This equates to a 0.5 FTE.

- **Nurses must have a solid and successful rating on their annual evaluation:** The purpose of this criterion was to ensure that nurses who participated in the program met their job requirements. Any nurses with a lower rating would not be eligible until they met the threshold of solid and successful.

- **Nurses must not have any active documented human resources corrective actions:** Again, this was to ensure that nurses who participated in the program were meeting job requirements.

## *Voluntary Versus Involuntary Participation*

The committee questioned the level of buy-in and motivation among nurses if their participation in the program was mandatory. So, we decided that participation in the program should be voluntary. We made this decision to leverage the program to empower nurses who were ready and eager to advance within their career and who were instilled with the drive and passion to positively influence our organization (CHMC, 2015). The clinical nurses on the committee strongly advocated this decision.

## *Levels of Achievement*

Determining how many levels the model should entail and calculating the threshold for each level was more challenging. Initially, the committee conceptualized four levels. However, trying to set parameters around four levels was difficult. Having four levels would also make the model more complicated to navigate. So, guided by the clinical nurses on the committee, who advocated for simplicity, we opted for two levels of achievement (CHMC, 2015):

- **Level 1:** This level would set the benchmark parameters of achievement.

- **Level 2:** This level would exceed these benchmark parameters.

Chapter 3 discusses each of these levels in more detail.

## *Framework to Showcase Achievement*

We needed to develop a framework for how nurses would demonstrate the successful completion of each level. Drawing from best practices we discovered during our search of the literature, we determined that each level would involve three categories (CHMC, 2015):

- **Clinical:** This category highlights the clinical advancement of the participant's nursing practice, demonstrated through positive outcomes.

- **Educational:** This category highlights the participant's educational advancement, demonstrated through professional development and knowledge sharing.

- **Professional:** This category highlights the participant's professional advancement, demonstrated through community, regional, and national involvement.

## *Activities*

We decided that various activities would be associated with each category (CHMC, 2015). Participants could complete these activities to demonstrate their proficiency and meet the benchmark parameters set for each level. These activities involved tasks above and beyond normal job expectations.

To foster autonomy, participants would be given the opportunity to choose from among a slate of activities for each category. This helped personalize the program for each participating nurse. The clinical nurses on the committee were essential in identifying activities that were above and beyond nurses' typical patient care role and that would showcase professional advancement.

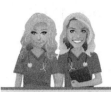

## GOOD IDEA

We based many activity requirements on standards for specific national recognition programs. This would enable our organization and our nurses to leverage our retention model to meet these national recognition standards and maintain national designations.

## *Objective or Subjective Measures*

As a committee, we needed to identify measures for gauging the success of each participant. First, though, we needed to determine whether the measures would be objective (fact-based), subjective (perception-based, including personal opinions), or both.

The committee opted for an objective review process, which required the use of objective measures and eliminating any bias (CHMC, 2015). This would result in a fair and standardized program in which all participating clinical nurses would be required to meet a consistent threshold to achieve level 1 or level 2 status. Taking an objective review approach also aligned with national recognition parameters to which our organization was accustomed.

To create an objective review process that would fairly measure the success of participating nurses, we needed to develop activities and requirements accordingly. This involved the following steps (CHMC, 2015):

- **Creating a model policy:** This policy outlined the program's overall purpose, process, and requirements. Having a policy was important for setting clear and concise expectations for nurses and nurse leaders.

- **Creating forms to confirm the authenticity of activities completed by participating nurses:** The most important element of each of these forms was a validator signature section to verify that nurses had in fact completed the activities they said they had.

- **Creating an explanation of activities document:** This document outlined all qualified program activities and associated requirements.

## Connecting With Key Organizational Objectives

Aligning the model with the organization's mission, vision, and strategies to ensure a return on investment was key to its sustainability. That meant ensuring that the outcomes achieved by participating nurses were measurable, quantifiable, and sustainable, and matched up with the organization's objectives. We also based many activity requirements on standards for specific national recognition programs to enable our organization and participating nurses to leverage the model to maintain national designations.

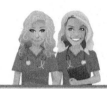 **MAKES SENSE**

To ensure program sustainability, we made sure to connect it with the value it would bring. If we could prove true value and return on investment through measurable outcomes, it would be hard to justify its dismantling down the line.

## Compensation

It wasn't just the organization's return on investment that mattered. We also needed to consider the return on investment for participating nurses—beyond developing professionally and embodying a career at the bedside. To that end, we developed a compensation package for nurses who successfully completed each level of the program (CHMC, 2015). This package was developed in close collaboration with human resources. Chapter 7 discusses the model's approach to compensation in more detail.

## *Nurse Autonomy*

The CNO and clinical nurses on the governing committee believed that nurse autonomy should be a key component of the model (CHMC, 2015). Nurse autonomy fosters professional development and pride in work completed. To meet this requirement, we worked to ensure that participating nurses could navigate the program easily and autonomously. Building a program that nurses could complete autonomously offered an additional benefit: The program could be self-sustainable and would therefore require less in the way of resources.

To promote nurse autonomy, the committee developed various resources for use by participating nurses. These included the following (CHMC, 2015):

- **An educational PowerPoint presentation:** Nurses would be required to view this presentation before applying for the program to ensure that they understood the program requirements and to set appropriate expectations. The presentation also helped increase transparency, promoted goal-setting among participants, and generated an overall sense of excitement about the program.

- **An explanation of activities document:** This document outlined all activities and requirements for both levels of the program. This was to help participating nurses identify what would be required of them to complete each of their chosen activities and to allow for an objective review process.

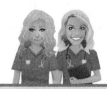

## *PRICELESS*

Leading, mentoring, and empowering nurses, rather than trying to manage their day-to-day activities—in other words, promoting nurse autonomy—does wonders to improve nurse retention and meet the organization's mission, vision, and strategic initiatives.

## Demonstrating Meeting Program Requirements

To determine how nurses should demonstrate that they had met program requirements, the committee explored options from the literature search. Ultimately, we decided that nurses should produce a portfolio (CHMC, 2015). This portfolio would showcase their outcomes for each chosen activity within each category. It would also enable them to methodically organize all their information and ensure an objective review process. As an added bonus, creating a portfolio would be a professional development activity in and of itself, which made our decision to take this approach that much easier.

## Program Frequency

Finally, the committee needed to determine the program's frequency— or more specifically, how frequently we would allow participating nurses to submit their portfolios. The committee tossed around many options:

- Anytime throughout the year

- Quarterly

- Twice per year

- Once per year

Due to sustainability considerations, we rejected the idea of accepting program submissions anytime throughout the year or quarterly (CHMC, 2015). Those options just weren't realistic—especially considering that at that time, we weren't sure who would facilitate the program. But accepting portfolio submissions just once per year seemed *too* infrequent. So, after a lot of collaboration and consideration, the committee chose to accept submissions twice per year (CHMC, 2015). This would allow enough time to review one round of portfolios before the next round was submitted and to deal with other aspects of the program, making it easier to facilitate and sustain the program. We selected April 1 and October 1 as our annual submission dates.

# IT'S ALL ABOUT THE LOOK

Once the details of the model were developed, it was time to create a brand for it—one that was meaningful and inspirational and that connected all the intentional elements woven throughout the program.

The committee decided that the model's brand should reflect the idea of one clinical nurse having a multifaceted organizational impact (CHMC, 2015). We then conducted brainstorming sessions to work out how to capture and convey this overall concept. We realized that the word *impact* seemed to encompass everything we wanted to express, so we homed in on that.

After deciding to focus on the word *impact*, we opted to turn it into an acronym that made the connections we wanted to highlight. Here's what we came up with:

- **Innovation:** Nurses innovate by thinking differently and putting into practice things that have not been done before. They refer to research, develop process improvements, and engage in evidence-based practices to ensure better care.

- **Mission driven:** Enabling nurses to connect to the organization's mission and vision empowers them to move strategic initiatives forward and expand their overall reach.

- **Patient centered:** Nurses are grounded in ensuring the delivery of high-quality care to patients and their families.

- **Advocate:** Nurses advocate for patients, families, and peers by supporting and promoting their best interests.

- **Collaboration:** Nurses collaborate with peers and other healthcare professionals as a team, using their unique perspectives, expertise, and education to solve patient care or healthcare system problems.

- **Thrive:** Nurses do all these things so the patients they serve can heal, grow, and thrive.

We brought this brand concept to marketing key stakeholders, who approved it. They then ran with our vision to formalize the model into a product (CHMC, 2016). Its official name became the IMPACT Recognition & Reward System, paraphrased as the IMPACT Model. Figure 2.1 shows the IMPACT Model logo, developed by the marketing team, and Figure 2.2 expands the IMPACT acronym.

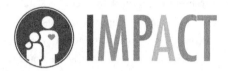

**FIGURE 2.1** IMPACT Model logo.

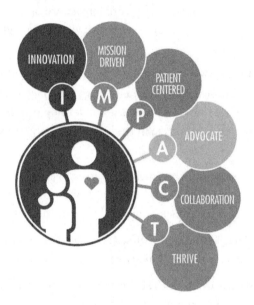

**FIGURE 2.2** IMPACT Model acronym.

## GETTING THE WORD OUT

Creating awareness and generating excitement about our new innovative model was crucial. About six months before our first portfolio submission date, the committee launched an awareness campaign. This involved putting posters in break rooms, generating email and newsletter articles, and so on (CHMC, 2015). We also asked our entire nursing leadership team to encourage clinical nurses within their area to apply.

This was crucial to the program's success. These nursing leaders were able to not only educate their clinical nurses about the model but also create connections across the enterprise for nurses interested in applying. The successful implementation of the IMPACT Model required a collective commitment by the entire nursing division.

# REFERENCES

Children's Hospital & Medical Center. (2015). *Children's Hospital & Medical Center.* Omaha, Nebraska.

Children's Hospital & Medical Center. (2016). *Children's Hospital & Medical Center.* Omaha, Nebraska.

*"This is where it all begins. Everything starts here, today."*

–David Nicholls

## CHAPTER 3

# IMPACT
# Model Overview

## INTRODUCTION

So how did we bring all those key decision points together to make a cohesive and operational program? We all know that going from a concept to an actual product can be a challenge. This was especially true with the IMPACT Model and all the multifaceted elements it entailed. Tying the elements together took great effort and methodical intention. This chapter outlines the overall framework of the IMPACT Model and how all of it came together. The next four chapters discuss each phase of the program in more detail.

## PURPOSE AND GOALS

A *purpose statement* explains why something exists. When creating the IMPACT Model purpose statement, we incorporated the IMPACT acronym to reflect the robust effect clinical nurses could have not only on themselves but also on their patients and the entire organization (Children's Hospital & Medical Center [CHMC], 2016).

Our purpose statement is as follows:

> To promote a career in direct patient care nursing through a formal recognition and reward program for nurses who demonstrate **innovation** in their nursing practice, in support of our **mission** through practicing **patient-centered** care, while participating in **advocacy** and **collaborating** so that all children **thrive** and are able to reach their full potential.

The IMPACT Model was developed with an overarching goal of positively influencing clinical nurse retention through empowerment and engagement, ultimately creating a career at the bedside. Retaining clinical nurses in their direct patient-care role positively influences many elements within a department. For example, it may result in:

- A robust mix of clinical skills and expertise within a team

- Better staffing standards to deliver safe patient care

- The development of trusting relationships between team members

- Overall cost savings, including reduced recruitment and orientation expenses

- A positive impact on a department's culture

Additionally, we wanted the IMPACT Model to produce an organizational impact. So, we also focused on improved organizational and patient outcomes that positively influenced the mission, vision, and strategic initiatives of the organization (CHMC, 2016).

Finally, we wanted to positively influence our organization's ability to meet standards and earn credentials and recognition from national programs such as the following (CHMC, 2016):

- American Nurses Credentialing Center (ANCC) Magnet Recognition Program®

- Commission on Accreditation of Medical Transport Systems Accredited Services

- American Association of Critical-Care Nurses Beacon Award for Excellence

- Extracorporeal Life Support Organization Award for Excellence

Placing clinical nurses in project-leadership roles and empowering shared decision-making with leadership and other disciplines are foundational aspects of many of these programs. We intentionally made these types of connections with the IMPACT Model so we could leverage our nurses' participation and outcomes as another return on investment.

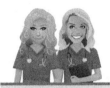

## SMART!

Recently, we were able to use 13 projects from the IMPACT Program in our effort to obtain recognition from a key national organization.

# IMPACT MODEL STRUCTURE

Any clinical nurse, inpatient or outpatient, within our enterprise may participate in the IMPACT Program. The target audience is clinical direct patient care nurses who spend at least 50% of their time working with patients. Eligible clinical nurses are also required to work a minimum of 20 hours (0.5 FTE), meet their basic job requirements, and have no documented incidences of corrective action by human resources (CHMC, 2015). As long as clinical nurses meet these program requirements, the number of years they have practiced as nurses is irrelevant.

The IMPACT Model consists of three phases, which span seven months on average. The phases are as follows:

- **Phase 1:** During this phase, nurses who might be interested in participating in the IMPACT Program learn about its requirements and expectations. They also make connections with key stakeholders to build a network of support.

- **Phase 2:** This is when nurses who choose to enroll in the IMPACT Program complete various activities to meet program requirements. These requirements fall into three program categories: clinical, educational, and professional. Participating nurses then complete a portfolio that showcases their achievements in each category.

- **Phase 3:** During this phase, nurses share their portfolio and are celebrated for their outcomes and accomplishments.

Chapters 4–7 describe these phases in greater detail.

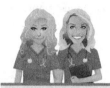

## SMART!

The IMPACT Model isn't just for nurses. It was created to be universal. When you're ready to expand, you can roll it out for any disciplines that have an impact on the organization's strategic initiatives.

# TWO LEVELS OF ACHIEVEMENT

The IMPACT Model supports two levels of achievement:

- **Level 1:** This level sets the standard parameters of achievement for the IMPACT Model.

- **Level 2:** This level exceeds the level 1 standard parameters with respect to expectations and the amount of work required.

Completion of both levels results in compensation. Nurses who complete level 2 receive a larger sum due to the additional work involved. Chapter 7 offers additional details on compensation.

# OVERALL REQUIREMENTS

The overall program requirements for both levels include the following (CHMC, 2015):

- Nurses must have a specialty certification to be eligible to participate in the program.

- Nurses must complete a specific number of continuing nursing education (CNE) hours to showcase their continued professional development. (This number differs depending on the program level.)

- Nurses must complete a project with outcomes that facilitate their professional development and positively contribute to the organization's mission, vision, and strategic initiatives.

- Nurses must complete a specific number of activities within each of the following categories:

  - Clinical

  - Educational

  - Professional

## Specialty Certification

All clinical nurses who want to participate in the IMPACT Program, whether in level 1 or level 2, must have a specialty certification approved by the ANCC (CHMC, 2015). Nurses who obtain a specialty certification demonstrate a commitment to lifelong learning and to their professional and leadership development. Evidence shows better patient outcomes due to increased knowledge and expertise and to continual learning through recertification (Williams & Counts, 2013).

### Specialty Certification Examples

- Certified Pediatric Nurse (CPN)

- Certified Diabetic Educator (CDE)

- Critical Care Nursing (CCRN)

- Certified Emergency Nurse (CEN)

- Oncology Certified Nurse (OCN)

## *Continuing Nursing Education (CNE) Hours*

Thanks to new evidence, research, technology, and so on, the field of healthcare is always evolving. Clinical nurses must keep up! They do this by participating in CNE (Staff writers, 2020).

All nurses must complete a specific number of CNE hours to maintain their registered nurse (RN) state licensure. In addition, nurses with specialty certification must complete CNE hours to obtain and maintain that certification.

Clinical nurses participating in the IMPACT Program are required to complete a minimum number of CNE hours. This number varies depending on which level they are pursuing. This is to demonstrate their commitment to professional development, which equips them to deliver high-quality patient care.

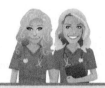

## *MAKES SENSE*

CNE courses that are required for your job, like Basic Life Support or Pediatric Advanced Life Support, don't count toward the IMPACT Program.

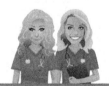

## *CHECK*

**Level 1 Requirements**
Minimum of 25 CNE hours

**Level 2 Requirements**
Minimum of 31 CNE hours

## *Project With Outcomes*

One main goal of the IMPACT Model is to be outcome-focused to help influence strategic initiatives and produce positive organizational outcomes. So, both levels of the model require participants to complete one project with measurable outcomes. This could be an evidence-based practice (EBP), a performance or process improvement (PI), or a relevant research project (CHMC, 2016).

The project needs to make sense from a strategic perspective, as well as with respect to the allocation of resources. For example, if a nurse chooses to work on an EBP project that is similar to one recently completed by a different nurse, the key stakeholders may require that nurse to come up with a different project.

Nurses must connect their projects with the organization's mission, vision, and strategic initiatives, and gather support for it from the right key stakeholders (CHMC, 2016). Stakeholders in our facility include:

- The nurse's direct supervisor

- Specific experts identified by the IMPACT committee

- For EBP projects, a clinical nurse specialist within the clinical education department who is an expert in EBP and facilitates the Nurse Residency and EBP Fellowship projects

- For PI projects, the nurse director of the performance improvement department

- For research projects, a clinical research RN who facilitates Research Fellowship projects

These leaders help ensure the IMPACT projects align with our strategies and are not a duplication of current or recent work.

After nurses choose a project, they must meet specific requirements. These differ from project to project and from level to level:

- For nurses on the level 1 track, the project and outcomes can be isolated within their department, and participating nurses can colead the project or actively participate.

- For nurses seeking to complete level 2, the project and outcomes must span the continuum, meaning they must involve the nurse's department and at least one other area, and participating nurses must lead or colead the project.

Other specific requirements differ depending on whether the project is an EBP, PI, or research project. These requirements are discussed in Chapter 6.

Both levels require participants to present their project to affected staff. This helps confirm that the participating nurse communicated with the right people about the project and effectively employed good change-management practices. It also serves as a professional development activity, which encourages participating nurses to work on leadership skills like public speaking, summarizing robust concepts, and explaining their work and outcomes in a clear and concise manner.

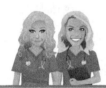

## *SIGN ME UP*

The IMPACT Model is intended for highly engaged nurses. Indeed, many of these nurses may already be "doing the work"—for example, an EBP, PI, or relevant research project. Indeed, this project might be well on its way to implementation and even measuring outcomes. Nurses may simply choose to formalize their efforts and outcomes through the IMPACT Program.

## *Category-Specific Activities*

As mentioned, the IMPACT Model involves three categories:

- Clinical

- Educational

- Professional

Each category is associated with specific activities that nurses must complete to showcase their proficiency and advancement. Some of these activities are required, while others may be selected as electives by the participating nurse (CHMC, 2015). Chapter 6 describes specific activities associated with each category.

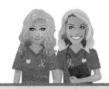

## SIGN ME UP

Nurses should choose activities with intention.

When nurses complete an activity, they earn activity points. Most activities count as 1 activity point; however, for some activities, nurses might earn more. For example, within the professional category, nurses can earn 1 activity point if they belong to a committee or council. However, if a nurse is a cochair or colead of the committee or council—a role that involves significantly more responsibility—he or she will be awarded 2 points.

In some cases, nurses can complete the same activity twice and earn activity points both times. For example, if nurses develop or update two policies, they can count both as activities for the clinical category. However, volunteering within the community can only count as 1 activity point—even if the nurse volunteers several times or for multiple organizations.

Some activities have a minimum time requirement. For example, the Enrichment Course activity, associated with the educational category, requires a minimum of four hours. This might involve one four-hour class, four one-hour classes, and so on. If multiple classes are involved, the participating nurse must provide evidence that she attended all sessions.

Clinical nurses participating in the IMPACT Program must earn a minimum number of activity points for each category. This number differs depending on which level they are pursuing.

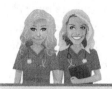

# CHECK

**Level 1 Requirements**

- **Clinical:** 3 activity points

- **Educational:** 3 activity points

- **Professional:** 3 activity points

**Level 2 Requirements**

- **Clinical:** 4 activity points

- **Educational:** 4 activity points

- **Professional:** 4 activity points

# REFERENCES

Children's Hospital & Medical Center. (2015). *Children's Hospital & Medical Center.* Omaha, Nebraska.

Children's Hospital & Medical Center. (2016). *Children's Hospital & Medical Center.* Omaha, Nebraska.

Staff writers. (2020). The nurse's continuing education toolkit. *Nurse Journal.* https://nursejournal.org/resources/nurses-continuing-education-guide/

Williams, H. F., & Counts, C. S. (2013). Certification 101: The pathway to excellence. *Nephrology Nursing Journal, 40*(3), 197–253.

# CHAPTER 4

# Phase 1:
# Where It All Starts

## INTRODUCTION

In Chapter 3, you learned that the IMPACT Model involves three phases. The purpose of phase 1 is to inform nurses about program requirements and expectations and to help them make connections with key stakeholders to develop a support network. This fosters professional growth and ensures that participating nurses' projects and outcomes will align strategically with the organization. This chapter outlines the various aspects of phase 1.

## GETTING ORGANIZED AND EDUCATED

When deciding whether to participate in the program, nurses must review an educational PowerPoint presentation that explains the details. This constitutes the official first step of phase 1. The educational PowerPoint presentation covers the following points:

- Why the model was developed

- Eligible nurses

- Compensation

- IMPACT Model policies

- Descriptions of all three phases

- Time frame requirements

- EBP, PI, and research project requirements

- Eligible activities

- Portfolio requirements

- Information about the IMPACT committee

- Presentation requirements

- The appeal process

- Who to contact with more questions

The PowerPoint presentation ensures program transparency. It also helps nurses determine whether they are qualified to participate in the program or to develop future goals to apply in the future.

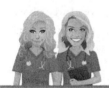

## MAKES SENSE

Participation in the IMPACT Program is voluntary. Nurses must actively pursue participation in the program. Simply choosing to participate is empowering in itself, as it requires nurses to work to develop the confidence to apply.

# UNDERSTANDING TIME FRAME PARAMETERS

The IMPACT Model involves various time frame parameters. The rationale behind these parameters is to ensure all activities completed are recent and relevant.

Some activities involve a minimum time frame. For example, nurses must be on a committee for a minimum of six months to earn activity points and include them in their portfolio. There is also a maximum time frame for activities. Specifically, all activities must be completed within 15 months of the April 1 or October 1 portfolio submission date. For example:

- If a nurse submits a portfolio on April 1, 2021, eligible portfolio content would include anything accomplished between January 1, 2020, and April 1, 2021.

- If a nurse submits a portfolio on October 1, 2021, eligible portfolio content would include anything accomplished between July 1, 2020, and October 1, 2021.

Any activities outside the 15-month time frame requirement would not be eligible for submission for the IMPACT Program.

# SUBMITTING A LETTER OF INTENT

Nurses who want to participate in the IMPACT Program and feel confident they meet the requirements must apply for the program. This involves completing a letter of intent. The purpose of the letter of intent—which is simply an electronic form the nurse fills out—is to inform the IMPACT committee that the nurse is interested in participating (Children's Hospital & Medical Center [CHMC], 2015). It is not a contract that *requires* the nurse to participate.

As shown in Figure 4.1, the letter of intent form is made up of several components. Some of these components relate to demographics. These include the following:

- Name

- Department

- Degree(s) held

- Years of nursing experience

- Years in current specialty area

Other components are meant to ensure that nurses are indeed able to participate in the IMPACT Program. These include:

- **Current specialty certification(s):** Nurses must have at least one.
- **Current full-time equivalent (FTE):** Nurses must be at least 0.5 FTE.

Additional components relate to the IMPACT Model itself. For example, nurses must disclose if they have ever submitted an IMPACT Model portfolio in the past (and if so, when), what level they are submitting for (level 1 or level 2), and the time frame in which they are planning to submit a portfolio (April or October). Finally, they must verify that they reviewed and understand the IMPACT Model educational PowerPoint and the program's policy.

IMPACT

Children's
HOSPITAL & MEDICAL CENTER

**Letter of Intent**

**Name/Credentials:** **Employee ID #:**

**Department:** **Years of Experience as an RN:** **Current FTE:**

**Years in Current Specialty:** **All Degree(s) Held:**

**Current Certifications:**

**Prior IMPACT Portfolio Submission** **(Month/Year)**

**Level Submitting for:** ☐ 1 ☐ 2

**Intended Portfolio Submission Date:** ☐ April ☐ October **Year:**

**I have reviewed and understand the IMPACT Education PowerPoint Presentation and Policy.** ☐ **Yes**

**RN Signature:** ______________________ **Date:**

**Required Criteria:**
- Clinical, direct patient care registered nurse
- Works a minimum of 0.5 FTE (20 hours/week)
- Solid & Successful on annual evaluation/six month if new employee
- No active disciplinary action greater than a documented discussion in file

______________________ ______________
Manager/Supervisor Signature Date

**Letter of Intent must be submitted at least four months prior to submission date:**
- Before June 1st for October submissions
- Before December 1st for April submissions

**FIGURE 4.1** Letter of intent.

A portion of the letter of intent must be filled out by the nurse's direct supervisor to verify that the nurse meets the IMPACT Model's eligibility requirements (CHMC, 2015). These include the following:

- The nurse is a clinical direct patient care nurse who works with patients at least 50% of the time.

- The nurse works at least 0.5 FTE (20 hours per week).

- The nurse received at least a "solid and successful" rating on her most recent annual review.

- The nurse has no corrective action beyond a documented discussion in his HR file.

This section warrants a discussion between the clinical nurse and the nurse's direct supervisor. The purpose of this discussion is to:

- Inform the supervisor of the nurse's desire to participate in the IMPACT Program

- Ensure the nurse meets all program eligibility requirements

- Allow the nurse to share details on the proposed EBP, PI, or relevant research project

- Enable the supervisor to match the nurse with expanded roles or special projects within the department or organization (if necessary)

After the clinical nurse completes the letter of intent—including the nurse supervisor section—the nurse submits it to the IMPACT committee. This is typically done by email. The letter of intent must be submitted at least four months before the nurse plans to submit a portfolio (CHMC, 2015).

- If the nurse plans to submit a portfolio on April 1, the letter of intent is due no later than December 1.

- If the nurse plans to submit a portfolio on October 1, the letter of intent is due by June 1.

However, nurses may submit a letter of intent before the four-month requirement if they choose. Submitting the letter of intent early enables nurses to set a proactive goal for all activities, project outcomes, and the completion of their portfolio.

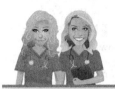

## MAKES SENSE

Successful participation in the IMPACT Program requires true intention and methodical planning. Last-minute submissions won't cut it!

The IMPACT committee compiles a list of all nurses who apply for the program. After the four-month submission deadline for letters of intent passes, the committee sends a welcome email to all nurses who qualify for participation and gives them the information and resources they need to complete the IMPACT Program.

# PROGRAM CONNECTIONS

At our facility, the IMPACT Model was intentionally connected with other programs designed to foster empowerment, engagement, and professional development (CHMC, 2016). These include the following:

- **The Nurse Residency Program:** This program is for new graduate nurses just entering the nursing field. It provides them with pointed pediatric training and ensures their competency to deliver safe pediatric patient care. Nurses in this program also complete an EBP project.

- **The EBP Fellowship and Research Fellowship programs:** These programs are geared toward experienced nurses who seek additional empowerment and professional development through the completion of EBP or research projects.

The IMPACT committee works collaboratively with leaders who facilitate these other programs to ensure there is synergy and consistency between them all (CHMC, 2016).

We encourage nurses who participate in these (and other) programs to consider the IMPACT Program, as they are already well on their way to completing an EBP or research project (CHMC, 2016). The IMPACT Model helps inspire these nurses to see their projects through implementation and to measure their impact via data-driven outcomes. The IMPACT Model also encourages these nurses to complete other activities within the organization or community, which further strengthens their engagement—and thus their retention.

Connecting the IMPACT Model with other programs has resulted in many positive outcomes. For example, before the development of the IMPACT Model, the Nurse Residency Program resulted in the implementation of only a few EBP projects. But since we connected the two programs, the implementation of projects from nurse residents has increased (CHMC, 2016).

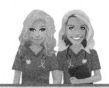

## MAKES SENSE

Any clinical nurse—inpatient or outpatient—who meets the qualifications to participate in the IMPACT Program can apply. This includes nurses who participate in these other programs as well as nurses who do not. However, nurses are not required to participate in other programs before or after applying for the IMPACT Program.

## REFERENCES

Children's Hospital & Medical Center. (2015). *Children's Hospital & Medical Center.* Omaha, Nebraska.

Children's Hospital & Medical Center. (2016). *Children's Hospital & Medical Center.* Omaha, Nebraska.

## CHAPTER 5

# Phase 2: How It Works

## INTRODUCTION

During phase 2 of the IMPACT Model, the clinical nurse develops a portfolio to showcase nursing excellence through activities and positive outcomes in the model's three categories: clinical, educational, and professional (Children's Hospital & Medical Center [CHMC], 2015). Developing the portfolio serves multiple purposes:

- It pulls all the activities and projects completed into one single deliverable.

- It represents a professional development opportunity because it requires nurses to create professional documents that showcase their achievements and outcomes.

- It ensures an objective review process to maintain the integrity of the IMPACT Model.

Nurses are expected to assemble their portfolio on their own. The information in this chapter illustrates how this is done.

# PORTFOLIO COMPONENTS

The portfolio developed by the clinical nurse in phase 2 must consist of the following components:

- Narratives
- Evidence
- Forms

## Narratives

In the narrative section of the portfolio, participating nurses tell their story by describing each of the activities they completed in paragraph form. These narratives empower the nurses to share their outcomes and achievements and enable the IMPACT committee to objectively assess whether the nurses met all program requirements (CHMC, 2015). Nurses should submit a separate narrative for each activity.

The nature of each narrative differs depending on what type of activity it describes. For example, the narrative for a community volunteering experience is different from a performance improvement project. In addition, some narrative requirements may differ depending on whether the nurse is on the level 1 track or the level 2 track because level 1 projects are implemented within one area, whereas level 2 projects must span the continuum.

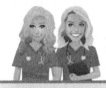

## KNOWLEDGE IS POWER

To determine what to include in each narrative, the nurse can refer to the explanation of activities document. This document is covered in more detail later in this chapter.

## *Evidence*

Nurses must submit their portfolio evidence of activities completed. This evidence supports and validates the information provided in the narrative section. This allows for an objective approach to the portfolio review process and helps to uphold the integrity of the IMPACT Model. The specific evidence submitted will be unique to each activity and is outlined in the explanation of activities document (discussed later in this chapter; CHMC, 2015).

## *Forms*

A series of forms were developed to include in the portfolio. These forms are key to ensuring the autonomous nature of the model. These include a portfolio planning form and various activity forms (CHMC, 2015).

A portfolio planning form is like a table of contents in a book. It outlines all the activities the nurse has chosen to showcase (CHMC, 2015). This form appears as the first page of the portfolio. The contents of this form will differ depending on whether the nurse is on the level 1 track or the level 2 track, as both levels have different requirements (see examples later in this chapter).

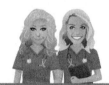 **MAKES SENSE**

The portfolio planning form is helpful for participating clinical nurses, as it acts as an overall road map of what they need to include in their portfolio.

In addition to the portfolio planning form, nurses must submit activity forms to describe any activities they completed. There are six types of these. The nurse must fill out one activity form for each activity completed. Each of these activity forms is placed at the beginning of the corresponding narrative to provide important details at a glance about the activity for the IMPACT committee (CHMC, 2015).

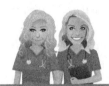

## CHECK

The activity forms are a little like face sheets used in healthcare. A *face sheet* is a one-page snapshot of a patient and his or her care.

The precise requirements of each of these activity forms differ in terms of information provided, but all of them call for the following:

- An activity title

- The dates the activity occurred (to ensure it was completed within the 15-month time frame)

- A validator signature (to confirm that the nurse in fact completed the activity in question—*not* whether the clinical nurse met IMPACT Model requirements)

For activity forms relating to evidence-based practice (EBP), process improvement (PI), and research projects, additional signatures are required, including from the nurse's direct supervisor, the nurse educator, and specific key stakeholders (which may differ depending on the type of project completed). The direct supervisor and nurse educator signatures confirm that the nurse received adequate support from department leaders for the project to be implemented and sustained, while the key stakeholder signatures verify that the nurse did not duplicate other projects. Figure 5.1 shows an example of an activity form (CHMC, 2015).

IMPACT

Children's
HOSPITAL & MEDICAL CENTER

**EBP | PI | Research Form Level 1**

**Applicant Name:**

**Clinical Activity:** (Must have an Evidenced-Based Project, Performance/Quality Improvement Project, or Research Project)

| | |
|---|---|
| **Evidenced-Based Project** | ☐ |
| **Performance Improvement** | ☐ |
| **Research Project** | ☐ |

**Project Title:**

**Project Dates:**

**Preapproved signatures required (prior to beginning project):**

**Clinical Educator/CNS** **Clinical Manager**

**EBP | PI | Research Leadership** **Applicant RN Signature**

**Validator Signature (Must be the Project Leader or Mentor)**
(As the validator you are attesting to the accuracy of the narrative written only, not the IMPACT Program requirements.)

**FIGURE 5.1** EBP, PI, & research activity form example.

# EXPLANATION OF ACTIVITIES DOCUMENT

The explanation of activities document (see Figure 5.2) outlines all qualified activities and their requirements. The explanation of activities document also outlines the number of activity points that can be achieved for each activity. Nurses can refer to this document to determine exactly what needs to be explained in each narrative, what evidence to submit, and which activity form applies for each activity. Nurses must meet all requirements of an activity outlined in the explanation of activities document for it to count (CHMC, 2015). Simply put, the IMPACT Program could not function without this document. It's the source of truth for the clinical nurse and the IMPACT committee.

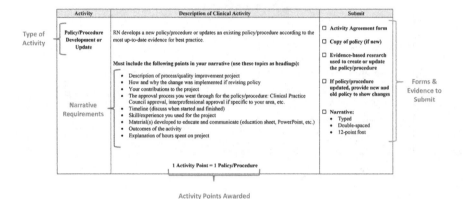

**FIGURE 5.2** Explanation of activities document example breakdown.

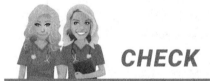

## CHECK

The explanation of activities document is the foundation of the entire IMPACT Model. It enables participating nurses to navigate the program independently and ensures an objective portfolio-review process.

The requirements for activities outlined in the explanation of activities document are the same for most—but not all—activities for nurses on the level 1 and level 2 tracks. The activities with differing requirements on these two tracks are the EBP, PI, and research projects. The most notable difference pertains to project scope. Nurses on the level 1 track can participate in or lead a project, and the outcomes can be isolated to their specific area. In contrast, nurses on the level 2 track must lead or colead the project, and the outcomes must apply to their own area and at least one other area within the organization to foster cross-continuum connection. This difference is reflected in the requirements for the portfolio narratives for each level (see Figures 5.3 and 5.4).

| Activity | Description of Clinical Activity (Level 1) | Submit |
|---|---|---|
| Evidence-Based Practice (EBP) Project | Must be preapproved (see EBP \| PI \| Research form)<br><br>RN had an active role in an EBP project using an EBP model (e.g., Johns Hopkins Nursing EBP Model, Iowa Model, etc.).<br><br>RN leads or co-leads an EBP project with a limited scope (e.g., impact on a single unit or narrow aspect of patient care on single unit).<br><br>Must include the following points in your narrative (use these topics as headings):<br><br>• Your role in EBP project<br>• Background to support project<br>• PICO question<br>• Collection and synthesis of evidence<br>• How the EBP project was implemented or communicated to specific area(s)<br>• EBP outcomes (or anticipated impact)<br> o What are your recommendations for change and your involvement in the implementation of change?<br> o What measures are in place to monitor sustainment of outcomes?<br> o If project ends in "no change" due to insufficient evidence or current practice is already evidence-based, please explain to receive activity points.<br>• Lessons learned<br><br>**1 Project with Active Role = 1 Activity Point**<br><br>**1 Project Lead/Co-lead = 2 Activity Points** | ☐ EBP \| PI \| Research form (Level 1)<br><br>☐ Literature Review table<br><br>☐ Benchmark table (if appropriate)<br><br>☐ PowerPoint report<br><br>☐ Education plan<br><br>☐ Any policy/procedures changed<br><br>☐ EBP project narrative:<br>• Typed<br>• Double-spaced<br>• 12-point font |

**FIGURE 5.3** Level 1 example for EBP project requirements.

| Activity | Description of Clinical Activity (Level 2) | Submit |
|---|---|---|
| Evidence-Based Practice (EBP) Project | Must be pre-approved (see EBP \| PI \| Research form)<br><br>RN leads or co-leads an EBP project using an EBP model (e.g., Johns Hopkins Nursing EBP Model, Iowa Model, etc.) with an impact across multiple areas.<br><br>Must include the following points in your narrative (use these topics as headings):<br><br>• Background to support project<br>• PICO question<br>• Collection and synthesis of evidence<br>• Recommendations to multiple areas/committees<br>• Use of interprofessional team to translate recommendations into practice<br>• Your role in EBP project<br>• How you collaborated, facilitated, and coordinated project across all areas impacted<br>• How the EBP project was implemented or communicated to specific areas<br>• EBP outcomes (or anticipated impact)<br>• Implementation of change<br>• Measures in place to monitor sustainment of outcomes/change<br> o Note: if project ends in "no change" due to insufficient evidence or current practice is already evidence-based, goes to a Level 1 submission<br>• Lessons learned<br><br>**1 Project = 4 Activity Points** | ☐ EBP \| PI \| Research form (Level 2)<br><br>☐ Literature Review table<br><br>☐ Benchmark table (if appropriate)<br><br>☐ PowerPoint report<br><br>☐ Education plan<br><br>☐ Any policy/procedures changed<br><br>☐ EBP project narrative:<br>• Typed<br>• Double-spaced<br>• 12-point font |

**FIGURE 5.4** Level 2 example for EBP project requirements.

As mentioned, the explanation of activities document also outlines the number of activity points clinical nurses can earn for each activity. This number differs depending on the amount of work involved (CHMC, 2015). For example, in the professional category, nurses who present outside our organization as an activity can earn 1 activity point if the presentation occurs at the local or state level or 2 activity points if the presentation occurs at the regional, national, or international level. This is because presenting in a regional, national, or international forum requires more in-depth work (see Figure 5.5).

| Activity | Description of Professional Activity | Submit |
|---|---|---|
| **Presentation Outside of Children's Hospital & Medical Center** | RN presents poster or lecture at a city, state, regional, national, or international conference or program.<br><br>**Must include the following points in your narrative (use these topics as headings):**<br><br>• Location presented and audience presented to<br>• The goals/objectives of the presentation<br>• How it benefited the target audience<br>• What you learned and what you would do different the next time<br>• Any potential next steps<br><br>┌─────────────────────────────────────────────┐<br>│ 1 Activity Point = Local or State Presentation │<br>│ 2 Activity Points = Regional, National, or International Presentation │<br>└─────────────────────────────────────────────┘ | ☐ **Presentation & Publications form**<br><br>☐ **Any handouts provided or picture of poster**<br><br>☐ **Narrative:**<br> • Typed<br> • Double-spaced<br> • 12-point font |

**FIGURE 5.5** Example of how activity points are earned depending on the extent of work completed by the clinical nurse.

# *OTHER PORTFOLIO REQUIREMENTS*

There are a few additional portfolio requirements (CHMC, 2016). These include the following:

- Narratives must be in 12-point font, double-spaced.

- Narratives must include headings that match the narrative requirements outlined in the explanation of activities document. This helps streamline the review process because it enables the IMPACT committee to easily match narrative requirements with the submitted narratives. It also makes it easier for nurses to ensure they meet all the requirements—a win-win.

- The portfolio must be presented in a three-ring binder with tabs or dividers to separate each narrative section.

- The portfolio must not use plastic sleeves. While plastic sleeves might make the portfolio look more professional, they make it harder for the IMPACT committee to scan it—something they do to keep a digital copy of each portfolio on file.

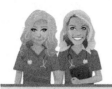

## *MAKES SENSE*

Keeping a copy of each portfolio prevents repeat participants from duplicating activities from a previous submission and ensures they complete new activities with new outcomes. It also helps when projects submitted for the IMPACT Program are used for national recognition renewals.

# *PUTTING IT ALL TOGETHER*

After the nurse has completed all narratives and forms, as well as compiled needed evidence, it's time to assemble the portfolio. The chronological order of the portfolio is as follows:

- Portfolio planning form

- Clinical activities, including the required forms, narratives, and evidence for each activity

- Educational activities, including the required forms, narratives, and evidence for each activity

- Professional activities, including the required forms, narratives, and evidence for each activity

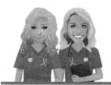

## *CHECK*

All portfolios must be in hard-copy form. Electronic portfolios are not accepted.

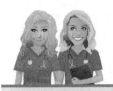

## GOOD IDEA

We encourage our nurses to get creative and personalize their port-folios by including personal photos and scrapbook-type elements. Personalizing is not required, however.

# PORTFOLIO SUBMISSION AND REVIEW

Nurses must submit their portfolios on or before April 1 or October 1. No late portfolio submissions are accepted. Typically, portfolios are dropped off outside a designated office in a dedicated receptacle. Nurses receive a confirmation email when the IMPACT committee receives their portfolio. The nurse must then wait to hear about next steps.

### What If I'm Late or Don't Complete the Program?

Some nurses might submit a letter of intent but fail to complete the necessary activities to submit a portfolio before the deadline (or at all). When this happens, these nurses are not subject to penalties or criticism. Members of the IMPACT committee understand that there may be many reasons a nurse does not submit a portfolio. For example, maybe the nurse needed more time to complete the project or collect the necessary outcomes. Or maybe the activities the nurse completed did not meet program requirements. Or perhaps the nurse just got too busy to commit the time needed to complete the program. Whatever the reason, there should be no pressure from the organization for the nurse to complete the program.

After the IMPACT committee reviews the nurse's portfolio, committee members decide, based on an objective review, whether the nurse has met all program requirements and should move on to phase 3 of the IMPACT Model. Nurses who do meet these requirements receive a congratulatory letter from the CNO. This letter also invites qualifying nurses to deliver a podium presentation highlighting their activities and outcomes on a specified date and time before an audience of peers and organizational leaders. Details of the podium presentation are highlighted in Chapter 7.

# *REFERENCES*

Children's Hospital & Medical Center. (2015). *Children's Hospital & Medical Center*. Omaha, Nebraska.

Children's Hospital & Medical Center. (2016). *Children's Hospital & Medical Center*. Omaha, Nebraska.

CHAPTER 6

# Portfolio Categories and Activities

## INTRODUCTION

You learned in Chapter 5 what is required for each participant's portfolio and how to assemble and submit it for the portfolio review process. However, you are probably wondering about the details on what activities are included in the IMPACT Model for nurses to select from, as Chapter 5 only provided a sneak peek. This chapter describes all the activities for each category so you can grasp the IMPACT Model entirely.

To further illustrate how to pull together all the activities completed for the program into a portfolio, and to highlight how the two levels are different, we've created sample portfolios for two pretend nurses, who we've named after ourselves—Judy and Mellisa. Pretend Judy is an inpatient clinical nurse applying for level 2, while pretend Mellisa is an outpatient nurse applying for level 1. These examples also showcase the autonomy of each nurse participating in pursuing and selecting activities they are passionate about.

# PORTFOLIO CATEGORIES AND ACTIVITIES

As you learned in Chapter 3, the IMPACT Program has specific requirements. These include the following:

- Having a specialty certification.

- Completing a minimum number of continuing nursing education (CNE) hours. (The specific number differs depending on whether you are applying for level 1 or level 2.)

- Completing an evidence-based practice (EBP), process improvement (PI), or research project with outcomes.

- Participating in a specific number of activities related to each category—clinical, educational, and professional. (Again, the specific number differs depending on whether you are applying for level 1 or level 2.)

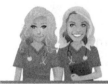

## CHECK

All activities for the IMPACT Model are organized into the clinical, educational, and professional categories.

## Clinical Category

Activities in the clinical category showcase clinical advancement of nursing practice, demonstrated through positive outcomes. Activities associated with the clinical category include the following (CHMC, 2015):

- **EBP project:** This is a project in which the nurse applies the best and most recent scientific research and evidence, combined with clinical expertise and patient values, to make decisions on how to deliver patient care that leads to improved outcomes (Conner, 2014). Many nurses complete EBP projects through the Nurse Residency Program for new graduate nurses and the EBP Fellowship program for experienced nurses. However, participating in one of these programs is not required to complete an EBP project for the IMPACT Program. Indeed, several nurses have completed an EBP project on their own. Activity points are awarded for EBP projects based on the IMPACT level for which the nurse is applying and how involved the nurse was with the project.

- **PI project:** This type of project involves reviewing a process or procedure, implementing changes, and measuring outcomes, with the goal of improving the process or procedure to better meet the needs of patients and staff (Conner, 2014). For example, a participating nurse might evaluate an inefficient process or one that frequently results in patient harm or near misses. Activity points are awarded based on the IMPACT level for which the nurse is applying and how involved the nurse was with the project.

- **Research project:** With this type of project, the nurse systematically studies materials and sources to establish facts and reach new conclusions (Conner, 2014). Most research projects submitted for the IMPACT Program have been completed through our facility's Research Fellowship program because completing a robust research project requires extensive knowledge, expertise, and the right key stakeholders. Activity points are awarded based on the IMPACT level for which the nurse is applying and how involved the nurse was with the project.

- **Policy or procedure development:** This involves developing a new policy or procedure or updating an existing one according to the most recent evidence to ensure best practice. Often, the policy or procedure nurses submit for the IMPACT Program relates to the EBP, PI, or research project they completed. Nurses can apply this activity as many as two times for a single portfolio submission.

- **Expanded role:** This involves participating in a role that goes above and beyond the nurse's normal job expectations without receiving extra compensation. Examples could include orienting new nurses to the organization, auditing, mentoring, acting as a super-user, and so on (see Figure 6.1). To earn 1 activity point, the nurse must perform the role for at least four hours in the 15-month time frame. Nurses can apply this activity as many as two times for a single portfolio submission.

| Activity | Description of Clinical Activity | Submit |
|---|---|---|
| **Expanded Role** | RN participates in an expanded role above and beyond the nurse's normal job expectations.<br><br>• Some applicable activities include, but not limited to: superuser, mentor, lead preceptor, auditor, donning/doffing leader, safety coach, and any role that is not receiving extra compensation.<br><br>**Must include the following points in your narrative (use these topics as headings):**<br><br>• Description of role<br>• How that role is above and beyond normal job expectations<br>• Purpose/objectives<br>• Timeline (discuss when started and finished)<br>• What skill/experience you used for this role<br>• Outcomes of the activity and how this role benefits Children's Hospital & Medical Center<br>• Explanation of hours spent on project<br><br>1 Activity Point = 4 hours minimum | ☐ **Activity Agreement form**<br><br>☐ **Narrative:**<br>• Typed<br>• Double-spaced<br>• 12-point font<br><br>☐ **Supporting document(s)** |

**FIGURE 6.1** Example of an activity in the clinical category.

- **Clinical special project:** This is a special project related to clinical aspects of patient care. Examples could include the development or update of an innovative process related to direct patient care, patient safety, nurse sensitive indicators, hospital-acquired conditions, and so on. To earn 1 activity point, the clinical nurse must spend at least four hours on the project in the 15-month time frame. Alternatively, the nurse can complete more than one project to meet the four-hour minimum requirement. Nurses can use this activity as many as two times for a single portfolio submission.

All nurses who participate in the IMPACT Program must complete either an EBP, a PI, or a research project to highlight organizational outcomes they helped produce. For nurses seeking to achieve level 2, this project will count as 4 activity points in the clinical category for either project they decide to pursue. For these nurses, no additional points are needed. Nurses seeking to achieve level 1 will receive 1–2 activity points in the clinical category. For an EBP or PI project, the nurse receives 1 activity point if they had an active role and 2 activity points if they led or coled. For a level 1 research project, the nurse receives 2 activity points, considering the amount of work a research project takes to complete. Level 1 nurses will need to complete additional activities to meet the requirements for this category.

## Clinical Category Activities

Let's see how Judy and Mellisa met the program requirements in the clinical category.

### Mellisa: Level 1 (3 Activity Points)

- **PI project:** Infusion Center FTE utilization improvement (1 activity point)

- **Policy update:** Rituxan (1 activity point)

- **Expanded role:** Auditor CLABI standardization (1 activity point)

### Judy: Level 2 (4 Activity Points)

- **EBP project:** Nurse-driven Foley removal algorithm (4 activity points)

## *Educational Category*

Activities in the educational category highlight advancement through professional development and knowledge sharing. These activities include the following:

- **CNE hours:** CNE activities are approved learning activities intended for professional development through education to enhance practice (Staff writers, 2020). For the IMPACT Model, completing a specific number of CNE hours (which differs by level) is a requirement and does not accrue activity points. Nurses must provide evidence of each CNE completed in their portfolio.

- **Evidence-based in-service or podium presentation:** Participating nurses must present one evidence-based in-service presentation via podium or poster to disseminate their EBP, PI, or research project (see Figure 6.2). This is mandatory. Presenting in a department-wide setting earns half an activity point (meaning nurses must present twice). Presenting at an organization-wide venue earns 1 activity point. Nurses can apply this activity as many as two times for the same portfolio submission.

| Activity | Description of Educational Activity | Submit |
|---|---|---|
| Evidence-Based Inservice or Podium Presentation | RN presents one evidence-based inservice or poster presentation based on current evidence.<br><br>**Must include the following points in your narrative (use these topics as headings):**<br><br>• The goals/objectives of the poster/presentation<br>• Who presented to<br>• Evidence used<br>• How it benefited the target audience<br>• What you learned and/or what you would do different next time<br>• Any potential next steps<br><br>**1 Activity Point = 2 Area/Department Presentations**<br>**or 1 Hospital Presentation** | ☐ Presentation & Publications form<br><br>☐ Supporting document(s)<br><br>☐ Narrative:<br>  • Typed<br>  • Double-spaced<br>  • 12-point font |

**FIGURE 6.2** Example of an activity in the educational category.

- **Educational special project:** This is a special project related to educational aspects of patient care or department/system operations. Examples could include teaching skills, educating on EBP, family support projects, and so on. To earn 1 activity point, nurses must spend at least four hours on the project in the 15-month time frame. Alternatively, they can complete more than one project to meet the four-hour minimum requirement. Nurses can apply this activity as many as two times for a single portfolio submission.

- **Instruction of certification course:** For this activity, nurses serve as an instructor for a healthcare-related certification course—for example, helping teach basic life support—above and beyond their job expectations. Nurses must teach at least two classes to earn 1 activity point. Nurses can apply this activity as many as two times for a single portfolio submission.

- **Enrichment course:** For this activity, participating nurses attend an educational course of their choosing to enhance their knowledge in their current area of practice. These courses need not be approved CNEs. At least four hours of coursework are required to earn 1 activity point. This can consist of a single four-hour course or multiple shorter courses. Proof of attendance must be submitted as evidence. Nurses can apply this activity as many as two times for a single portfolio submission.

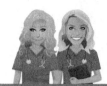

## *MAKES SENSE*

Nurses cannot count the CNE courses required for level 1 and level 2 status as enrichment courses. Different education courses must be used for this activity.

- **Healthcare academic course:** For this activity, participating nurses complete a nursing-related academic course— that is, a course in a nursing degree program or taken for academic credit. The nurse must earn a grade of B or higher or pass if the course is pass/fail. Three credit hours (whether earned from a single course or multiple courses) equals 1 activity point. Nurses can apply this activity as many as two times for a single portfolio submission.

- **Presentation within the organization:** For this activity, participating nurses deliver a presentation to educate staff within the organization on a relevant topic. Presentation content need not be evidence-based. Presenting in a department-wide setting earns half an activity point (meaning nurses must present twice). Presenting at an organization-wide venue earns 1 activity point. Nurses can apply this activity as many as two times for a single portfolio submission.

## Educational Category Activities

Let's see how Judy and Mellisa met the program requirements in the educational category.

### Mellisa: Level 1 (3 Activity Points)

- **CNEs:** 25

- **PI presentation:** Two Infusion Center staff meetings (1 activity point)

- **Enrichment course:** Hunter syndrome presentation (1 activity point)

- **Enrichment course:** Xatmep medication presentation (1 activity point)

### Judy: Level 2 (4 Activity Points)

- **CNEs:** 32.75

- **EBP presentation:** One PICU staff meeting (1 activity point)

- **EBP presentation:** One med-surg staff meeting (1 activity point)

- **Healthcare academic course:** Nursing 722: Child Care Management (1 activity point)

- **Enrichment course:** Pediatric surgical services conference (1 activity point)

## *Professional Category*

Activities in the professional category demonstrate advancement through community, regional, and national involvement in professional pursuits. These activities include the following:

- **Specialty certification:** A specialty certification demonstrates a commitment to advanced knowledge and expertise in a defined functional or clinical area of nursing (Williams & Counts, 2013). For the IMPACT Program, having at least one specialty certification—for example, Critical Care Registered Nurse or Certified Pediatric Nurse certification—is considered a foundational element and therefore does not count toward an activity point. Nurses must submit proof of certification in their portfolio.

- **Additional specialty certification:** For this activity, nurses earn a second specialty certification approved by the American Nurses Credentialing Center. This additional certification counts as 1 activity point. Nurses who are triple-certified can apply this activity as many as two times for a single portfolio submission.

- **Membership in a professional organization:** Nurses can earn 1 activity point for being an active member in a nursing professional organization, such as the American Nurses Association (see Figure 6.3). Being a member of a professional nursing organization enables nurses to learn about the latest research and evidence, improve their clinical skills, and grow their professional network (Greggs-McQuilkin, 2005). This activity can be applied only one time for a single portfolio submission.

| Activity | Description of Professional Activity | Submit |
|---|---|---|
| Professional Organization Membership | RN has been an active member of a nursing professional organization for at least six months. <br><br> **Must include the following points in your narrative (use these topics as headings):** <br><br> • Member for at least six months during the 15-month submission time (must include year and/or months). <br> • Describe the meetings attended or the activities in which you are involved. <br> • Why are you a member and how does it benefit you? <br> • If you hold an organization officer position, please describe your roles and responsibilities, including dates of involvement and the contact information of a committee member. <br><br> **1 Activity Point = Membership** <br><br> **2 Activity Points = Organization Officer** <br><br> (This activity can only be used one time.) | ☐ **Professional Organization form** <br><br> ☐ **Copy/verification of membership attached with year/months** <br><br> ☐ **Narrative for professional organization membership:** <br> • Typed <br> • Double-spaced <br> • 12-point font |

**FIGURE 6.3** Example of an activity in the professional category.

- **Publication:** This activity involves contributing to a publication such as an academic journal, book, and so on. This type of activity can be time-consuming, so one publication equates to 2 activity points. Nurses can apply this activity as many as two times for a single portfolio submission if they are published in two separate publications.

- **Membership on a committee/council:** Nurses can earn activity points by being an active member of a department, hospital, or system committee or council, such as a shared professional governance council/committee, a Hospital Acquired Conditions (HAC) committee, and so on. Activity points are awarded based on the nurse's level of involvement. Being an active member of a committee/council earns 1 activity point; serving as a co-chair earns 2 activity points due to the additional work involved. Nurses can apply this activity as many as two times for a single portfolio submission if they participate in two different committees/councils.

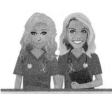

## *MAKES SENSE*

Nurses must have been a member of a committee/council for at least six months during the 15-month program time frame before submitting their portfolio. This is to ensure the nurse is in fact an active member of the committee/council and did not join simply for the purposes of the IMPACT Program.

- **Presentation outside of organization:** For this activity, the nurse presents a poster or podium lecture at a local, state, regional, national, or international conference, forum, or program. Activity points are awarded based on the event type. Presenting at a local or state event earns 1 activity point; presenting at a regional, national, or international event earns 2 activity points. Nurses can apply this activity as many as two times for a single portfolio submission if they present at two different events.

- **Community volunteering:** For this activity, the nurse volunteers in the community for a health- or non-health related organization, without receiving compensation. At least six hours of volunteering are required to earn 1 activity point. This can consist of a single six-hour volunteer shift or multiple shorter shifts. This activity can be applied only one time for a single portfolio submission.

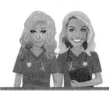

## *MAKES SENSE*

All volunteer activities must be preapproved by the IMPACT committee.

- **Professional special project:** This activity involves the completion of a special project related to patient care, professional practice, or department/system operations—for example, inventing a process that results in cost savings, time savings, productivity improvement, and so on. To earn 1 activity point, nurses must spend at least four hours on the project in the 15-month time frame. Alternatively, they can complete more than one project to meet the four-hour minimum requirement. Nurses can apply this activity as many as two times for a single portfolio submission.

## Professional Category Activities

Let's see how Judy and Mellisa met the program requirements in the professional category.

### Mellisa: Level 1 (3 Activity Points)

- **Specialty certification:** Certified Pediatric Nurse

- **Additional certification:** Chemotherapy and biotherapy provider (1 activity point)

- **Membership in professional organization:** President of the Association of Hematology & Oncology Nurses (2 activity points)

### Judy: Level 2 (4 Activity Points)

- **Specialty certification:** Certified Pediatric Nurse

- **Additional certification:** Critical Care Registered Nurse (1 activity point)

- **Membership on committee:** PICU HAC Group (1 activity point)

- **Membership in professional organization:** American Association of Critical-Care Nurses (1 activity point)

- **Volunteer:** Meals on Wheels (1 activity point)

## The Portfolio Planning Form

Let's see what Judy's and Mellisa's portfolio planning forms look like. Figure 6.4 shows Judy's form, and Figure 6.5 shows Mellisa's. Notice the differences between the level 1 and level 2 forms.

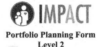 

**Portfolio Planning Form**
**Level 2**

**Name/Credentials: Judy Thomas, BSN, RN, CCRN, CPN**

**Submission Date: 04/01/2021**

| | |
|---|:---:|
| **CLINICAL**<br>Must have an EBP, PI, or Research activity that impacts across the continuum of care<br>(Another area has been educated on the topic for potential/actual implementation) | ☑ |
| 1. <u>**EBP Project: Nurse-Driven Foley Removal Algorithm**</u> | |
| **EDUCATIONAL**<br>Four activities in at least three areas + at least 31 contact hours/year<br>(Must have an activity where you educated beyond your area a change in practice in which<br>you played a key role in dissemination of knowledge) | ☑ |
| Number of Contact Hours: **32.75** | |
| 1. <u>**EBP Presentation: Nurse-Driven Foley Removal Algorithm to**</u><br><u>**PICU Staff**</u> | |
| 2. <u>**EBP Presentation: Nurse-Driven Foley Removal Algorithm to**</u><br><u>**Five Med-Surg Staff**</u> | |
| 3. <u>**Healthcare Academic Course: Nursing 722 Childcare**</u><br><u>**Management**</u> | |
| 4. <u>**Enrichment Course: Pediatric Surgical Service Conference**</u> | |
| **PROFESSIONAL**<br>Four activities in at least three areas + Specialty Certification<br>(Volunteer and professional organization membership can only be used once) | ☑ |
| Specialty Certification: **CPN** | |
| 1. <u>**Additional Certification: CCRN**</u> | |
| 2. <u>**Committee Council: PICU HAC Committee**</u> | |
| 3. <u>**Professional Organization Membership: AACN**</u> | |
| 4. <u>**Community Volunteer: ENOA Meals on Wheels**</u> | |

**FIGURE 6.4** Example of a completed level 2 portfolio planning form.

*Continued*

## The Portfolio Planning Form *Continued*

**Portfolio Planning Form**
**Level 1**

Applicant Name/Credentials: **Mellisa Renter, BSN, RN, CPN**

Submission Date: **04/01/2021**

| | |
|---|:---:|
| **CLINICAL**<br>Three activities in at least two areas<br>(Must have an EBP, PI, or Research activity) | ☑ |
| 1. PI: Infusion Center FTE Utilization Improvement | |
| 2. Policy/Procedure Development: Rituxan | |
| 3. Expanded Role: Auditor CLABSI Standardization | |
| **EDUCATIONAL**<br>Three activities in at least two areas + at least 25 contact hours/year<br>(Must have an evidence-based inservice or podium presentation) | ☑ |
| Number of Contact Hours: **25** | |
| 1. Podium Presentation: Infusion Center FTE Utilization | |
| 2. Enrichment Course: Hunters Syndrome Presentation | |
| 3. Enrichment Course: Xatmep Medication Presentation | |
| **PROFESSIONAL**<br>Three activities in at least two areas + Specialty Certification<br>(Volunteer and professional organization membership can only be used once) | ☑ |
| Specialty Certification: **CPN** | |
| 1. Additional Certification: Chemotherapy and Biotherapy Provider | |
| 2. Professional Organization Membership: Association of Hematology Oncology Nurses – President | |
| 3. Professional Organization Membership: Association of Hematology Oncology Nurses – President | |

**FIGURE 6.5** Example of a completed level 1 portfolio planning form.

# Congratulations! You've Advanced to Phase 3!

Figures 6.6 and 6.7 show the congratulatory letters Judy and Mellisa received following their portfolio submission and review.

Children's
HOSPITAL & MEDICAL CENTER

Judy Thomas, BSN, RN, CCRN, CPN

Thank you for your interest in the IMPACT Reward and Recognition Program at Children's Hospital & Medical Center. Your commitment to continue your clinical growth, professional development, and promotion of excellence in patient care is evident through the portfolio you submitted.

I am pleased to let you know that you have successfully met the initial requirements for the IMPACT Program Level 2 for April 2021. For the next step, please plan to present your portfolio information on **Tuesday, June 14**[th], in the Glow Auditorium. Please arrive no later than 10:00 a.m.; the program will finish by 11:30 a.m. You will be receiving an email with the requirements regarding the presentation.

As the CNO/COO of Children's Hospital & Medical Center, I want to extend my gratitude for all you do and personally congratulate you on this remarkable achievement.

*Kathy English*

Kathy English, MSN, MBA, RN, FACHE
Executive Vice President,
Chief Nursing Officer, &
Chief Operations Officer

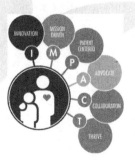

8200 Dodge Street | Omaha, NE 68114-4113 | 402-955-5400 | ChildrensOmaha.org

**FIGURE 6.6** Sample congratulatory letter to advance to phase 3.

*Continued*

## Congratulations!
## You've Advanced to Phase 3! *Continued*

Mellisa Renter, BSN, RN, CPN

Thank for your interest in the IMPACT Reward and Recognition Program at Children's Hospital & Medical Center. Your commitment to continue your clinical growth, professional development, and promotion of excellence in patient care is evident through the portfolio you submitted.

I am pleased to let you know that you have successfully met the initial requirements for the IMPACT Program Level 1 for April 2021. For the next step, please plan to present your portfolio information on **Tuesday, June 14th,** in the Glow Auditorium. Please arrive no later than 10:00 a.m.; the program will finish by 11:30 a.m. You will be receiving an email with the requirements regarding the presentation.

As the CNO/COO of Children's Hospital & Medical Center, I want to extend my gratitude for all you do and personally congratulate you on this remarkable achievement.

*Kathy English*

Kathy English, MSN, MBA, RN, FACHE
Executive Vice President,
Chief Nursing Officer &
Chief Operations Officer

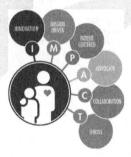

8200 Dodge Street  |  Omaha, NE 68114-4113  |  402-955-5400  |  ChildrensOmaha.org

**FIGURE 6.7** Sample congratulatory letter to advance to phase 3.

# *REFERENCES*

Children's Hospital & Medical Center. (2015). *Children's Hospital & Medical Center.* Omaha, Nebraska.

Conner, B. T. (2014, June 11). Differentiating research, evidence-based practice, and quality improvement. *American Nurse Journal.* https://www.myamericannurse.com/differentiating-research-evidence-based-practice-and-quality-improvement/

Greggs-McQuilkin, D. (2005). Why join a professional nursing organization? *Nursing, 35*(19).

Staff writers. (2020). The nurse's continuing education toolkit. *Nurse Journal.* https://nursejournal.org/resources/nurses-continuing-education-guide/

Williams, H. F., & Counts, C. S. (2013). Certification 101: The pathway to excellence. *Nephrology Nursing Journal, 40*(3), 197–253.

*"It had long since come to my attention that people of accomplishment rarely sat back and let things happen to them. They went out and happened to things."*

–Leonardo Da Vinci

## CHAPTER 7

# Phase 3: Presenting, Recognizing, and Celebrating

## INTRODUCTION

The final phase of the IMPACT Model is phase 3. During phase 3, all nurses who met all IMPACT Model requirements in the most recent round of portfolio submissions gather to share their achievements and outcomes before an audience of organizational leaders and peers. They do this by way of a PowerPoint presentation. Delivering this presentation is required to successfully complete phase 3.

The purpose of the PowerPoint presentation is threefold:

- To disseminate each nurse's findings during the course of the IMPACT Program

- To provide nurses who participated in the program with one last professional development opportunity

- To recognize and celebrate the achievements of all nurses who completed the program

This chapter discusses phase 3 of the IMPACT Model in more detail.

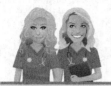

## MAKES SENSE

Nurses must complete phase 3 to be eligible for compensation.

# PUTTING TOGETHER THE PRESENTATION

A week or so after participating nurses receive the congratulatory letter from the CNO indicating that they successfully completed phase 2 of the IMPACT Program and inviting them to advance to phase 3, the IMPACT committee sends an email to the nurses outlining next steps. This email:

- Confirms that these nurses have been invited to advance to phase 3

- Outlines presentation requirements

- Indicates who will attend the presentation ceremony (more on this in the next section)

As far as presentation requirements go, each presentation should include the following:

- **A brief bio of the presenting nurse:** This should include the nurse's title, the department in which the nurse works, how many years the nurse has been practicing, and how long the nurse has been with our organization.

- **A high-level overview of activities completed:** This should include all activities completed in the clinical, educational, and professional categories.

- **An in-depth review of the nurse's evidence-based practice, process improvement, or research project:** This should include why the nurse chose that particular project, how the nurse progressed from project launch to implementation, and how project outcomes positively influenced the organization.

- **Why the nurse chose to participate in the IMPACT Program:** The nurse should also note how the program helped her grow professionally and why the program is important to her and to the organization.

Typically, the presentation ceremony occurs six to eight weeks after participating nurses receive the congratulatory letter from the CNO. During this time, these nurses develop their PowerPoint presentations. To aid with this, the IMPACT committee provides a presentation template. This streamlines the development process and helps nurses ensure that all required elements are included.

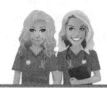

## GOOD IDEA

Although some nurses have experience developing and delivering PowerPoint presentations, others do not. Nurses who have questions while developing their PowerPoint presentation should turn to the IMPACT committee for help.

Presentations are due to the IMPACT committee one week before the presentation ceremony. This is to ensure that the committee receives all presentations on time. It also enables the committee to review each presentation to ensure they include all required elements. If anything is missing from a nurse's presentation, the committee works with that nurse to make sure any necessary adjustments are made.

> ### What Should You Wear?
>
> What should participating nurses wear to the presentation ceremony? It depends on the nurse. Some nurses like to dress up—especially if the presentation ceremony is on their day off. However, nurses who are working on the day of the presentation might attend in their scrubs. The bottom line? As long as your clothes adhere to the organization's dress code, you're fine.

# TIME TO BRAG: PRESENTING PORTFOLIO OUTCOMES

At Children's, we conduct our IMPACT Program presentation ceremony in the auditorium. Before the presentations begin, members of the IMPACT committee take the stage to provide a brief overview of the program, explain why it exists, and outline the outcomes it has produced. Then the committee introduces each nurse one by one to deliver their presentations. Nurses deliver their presentations from a podium on the stage, with their PowerPoint slides displayed behind them. Each nurse has about 20 minutes to present.

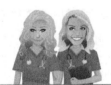 *SMART!*

> Recently, we added a virtual option to include attendees who are unable to join in person.

Each presentation ends with a Q-and-A session. This allows audience members to make comments or ask questions. Comments often relate to how much of an impact (no pun intended) the nurse's achievements and outcomes have made on the organization. Questions usually pertain to next steps, how the project could be expanded, whether nurses plan to publish or present their findings at a conference, and so on.

## The Audience

Attendance at the presentation ceremony is typically robust, especially among executives. Presentation attendees typically include the following people:

- The chief nursing officer
- The chief executive officer
- The chief medical officer
- The senior vice president of human resources
- Nurse directors
- Nurse managers
- Clinical nurse specialists
- Nurse educators
- Clinical nurses
- Other nurses throughout the organization
- Providers

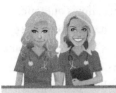

## MAKES SENSE

Because we have two portfolio submission dates per year, we hold two presentation ceremonies in that same time frame.

# LET'S CELEBRATE!

After all the nurses finish their presentations, the forum shifts to a celebration. To kick off the celebration, members of the IMPACT committee congratulate the nurses for their achievements and thank them for their contributions. We also offer a quick overview of the program's purpose, its impact on nurse retention, projects completed by participating nurses so far, and so on. Then the CNO takes the stage to offer words of inspiration and praise for participating nurses and for the IMPACT Program as a whole. Nurses are then called to the stage one at a time to receive their IMPACT Program certificate of recognition and a bouquet of flowers and to be photographed with the CNO. After that, the participating nurses assemble for a group picture. Finally, members of the IMPACT committee thank everyone for attending and recognize participating nurses one last time for all their work.

## Certificates of Recognition

Figures 7.1 and 7.2 show the certificates of appreciation for pretend Judy and pretend Mellisa.

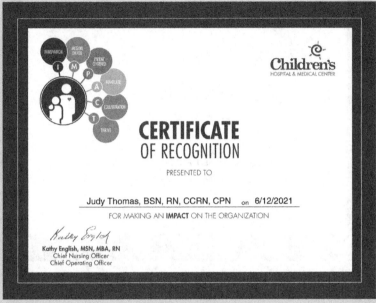

**FIGURE 7.1** Example of IMPACT Program certificate.

*Continued*

**Certificates of Recognition** *Continued*

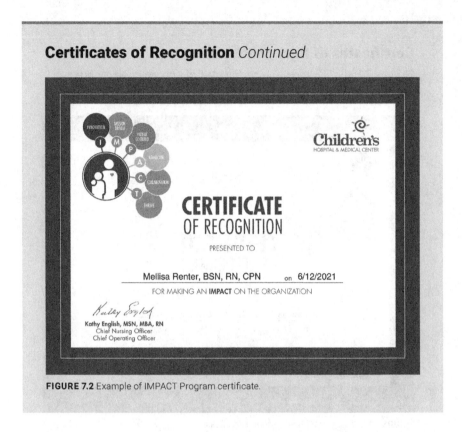

**FIGURE 7.2** Example of IMPACT Program certificate.

# ORGANIZATIONAL INVESTMENT: COMPENSATION

After successfully completing all phases and meeting all requirements of the IMPACT Program, nurses will automatically begin receiving the associated compensation—*if* they remain clinical nurses who work with patients at least 50% of the time. Only nurses who continue in this role will be compensated in full. This helps improve nurse retention.

Organizations must realize the importance of investing in current staff to drive engagement and retention. This includes making monetary investments—for example, compensating clinical nurses who devote time to completing programs (like the IMPACT Program) that result in positive organizational outcomes.

To receive full compensation for completing the IMPACT Program, nurses must do the following:

- Successfully complete a portfolio in phase 2 and present it in phase 3

- Remain a clinical nurse for one year after completing the program

After nurses complete phase 3 of the IMPACT Program, they receive compensation on a quarterly basis over the course of one year—*if* they meet additional eligibility requirements. Specifically, the nurse must:

- Be employed within the organization as a clinical nurse at the end of each quarter

- Maintain a job status of at least a 0.5 FTE (20 hours per week)

- Receive a solid and successful rating on their annual evaluation

- Receive no corrective action from human resources during the payout time frame

No doubt you're wondering how much nurses are paid to complete the IMPACT Program. Well, it depends on what level they achieve:

- **Level 1:** Compensation for level 1 is $5,000, paid in four installments of $1,250 over the course of one year.

- **Level 2:** Compensation for level 2 is $10,000, paid in four installments of $2,500 over the course of one year.

This might sound like a lot of money—more than your organization's budget can allow. But consider that, on average, between $5.2 million to $8.0 million is lost annually due to bedside nurse turnover (Vaughn, 2020).

The expenses involved with the IMPACT Program are pennies compared to that. Indeed, spending in this way can actually save your organization money.

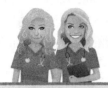

## SMART!

We designed the compensation program with the intention to improve retention and drive other positive outcomes.

As for the disbursal of payments, we add them to the last paycheck of each quarter—*after* the IMPACT committee verifies with the nurse's supervisor that the nurse has met eligibility requirements. Once the committee verifies the nurse's eligibility, they notify the HR department, which releases the payment.

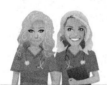

## MAKES SENSE

If a nurse moves from a bedside role before the one year is up, compensation will be prorated accordingly.

The IMPACT Program compensation package for each participating nurse, regardless of level, also includes a discretionary fund of $1,000. These funds are meant to be used to cover educational and professional advancement expenses, such as the following:

- License renewal

- Conference attendance

- Professional books or journals

- Professional organization memberships

- Educational courses

Participating nurses must use discretionary funds within one year of finishing phase 3 of the IMPACT Program. They must also meet the aforementioned eligibility requirements.

When it comes to their discretionary fund, nurses must "use it or lose it." If nurses don't use all $1,000 of the discretionary fund within the one-year time frame, they will not receive whatever amount is left over.

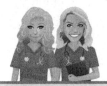

## MAKES SENSE

Don't leave funds on the table! Nurses should start thinking about how they want to spend their discretionary fund as early as possible.

Discretionary funds are distributed retroactively. That is, participating nurses must cover the educational or professional advancement expense upfront. They will then be reimbursed. To ensure reimbursement, we *strongly* suggest that participating nurses obtain approval for the expense from the director of professional nursing practice beforehand to make sure it meets the criteria for reimbursement.

We find that the discretionary funds offer a real return on investment—not just for our nurses, but for the organization as a whole. For example, suppose a nurse uses these discretionary funds to attend a conference, where he learns new best practices or encounters an innovative idea to improve a key process. The nurse then brings these findings back to the organization—and brings the investment full circle. The findings may also serve as the foundation for a new project for the nurse's next IMPACT Program portfolio, which could have a positive impact on the broader organization. As an organization, we have also found that we can leverage our nurses' professional development experiences, paid for by these discretionary funds, to achieve our national designations—yet another return on investment. The possibilities are endless when you empower clinical nurses to pursue their professional interests. You invest in them, and they invest in you.

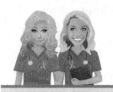

# PRICELESS

While the compensation package is important, we have found that most nurses do not participate in the IMPACT Program just for the money. They get so much more than the financial reward!

## WHAT'S NEXT?

Additional next steps will differ depending on the clinical nurse and his project. These steps may include:

- Expanding the project to other areas within the organization

- Presenting at other organizational forums to share outcomes

- Publishing or presenting at a conference

A lot of participants who complete level 1 of the IMPACT Model roll right into completing level 2—choosing a new project and activities. Others simply pursue new opportunities to positively affect their department or the organization as a whole. Really, with a program like IMPACT in place to ignite their passion, the sky is the limit on what these clinical nurses can achieve!

## REFERENCE

Vaughn, N. (2020, October 27). *Nurse turnover rates: How to reduce healthcare turnover*. https://www.relias.com/blog/how-to-reduce-healthcare-turnover

## CHAPTER 8

# Program Leadership: The IMPACT Committee

## INTRODUCTION

There is nothing more frustrating than spending time, money, and resources to create a new program or launch a new initiative only to watch it crumble right before your eyes. One main reason new programs and initiatives collapse is because their facilitators fail to follow the plan-do-check-act model. Sure, they do well with the planning and doing. But when it comes to checking how the program is going and acting on program outcomes, not so much. We were *not* going to let that happen with the IMPACT Program.

Before we rolled out the IMPACT Model, we needed a clear understanding of who would be accountable for identifying what was and was not working, updating and enhancing as needed, and ensuring our guiding principles were being followed and our intended outcomes were being met. To that end, we created the IMPACT committee. This chapter covers the roles and responsibilities of IMPACT committee members.

# WHO SERVES ON THE IMPACT COMMITTEE?

Deciding who should serve on the IMPACT committee involved answering a few key questions:

- Would the committee consist of organizational leaders?

- Should committee membership include clinical nurses, and if so, how should they be involved?

- How many leaders and staff would be needed to ensure a consistent and objective approach to the program?

Initially, we took a "more is better" approach. When the IMPACT Model rolled out, the committee included eight members—a mix of clinical nurses, supervisors, and directors, and the SVP of HR (Children's Hospital & Medical Center [CHMC], 2015). We quickly realized, however, that this committee structure posed a few problems. First, keeping all eight committee members moving in the same direction was challenging, to say the least. Second, our more senior committee members sometimes grappled with maintaining objectivity about their staff who applied or participated in the program. And third, the clinical nurses on the committee:

- Had little time to commit to the program

- Struggled with mentoring their peers on the committee as they worked in different units or areas

- Sometimes had trouble being fair and objective regarding their peers

- Were unsure how to navigate the tension between participating in the program and remaining objective as committee members

In response, we agreed to take an entirely new approach to the committee. We pared it down to two program leaders (that would be us) in partnership with the CNO and SVP of HR (CHMC, 2016). As program leaders, we do have other responsibilities within the organization, but we have no direct reports who are eligible to participate in the program. This was an objective approach.

# IMPACT COMMITTEE RESPONSIBILITIES

Members of the IMPACT committee—especially the two program leaders—have several responsibilities to operationalize and safeguard the program. These include the following (CHMC, 2016):

- Evaluating the IMPACT Model
- Conducting meetings
- Mentoring support
- Reviewing portfolios
- Handling appeals
- Planning the presentation ceremony
- Dealing with compensation

## Evaluating the IMPACT Model

At least once a year, we review and revise IMPACT Model policies, procedures, and requirements to ensure that the program continues to meet its guiding principles. This review considers feedback from clinical nurses (provided during mentoring sessions) and from leadership, as well as lessons learned during the portfolio review process (discussed later in this chapter).

## Conducting Meetings

Seriously, we do *not* need more meetings added to our calendar! So, we don't conduct regular meetings. Rather, we schedule them only as needed (and only if a quick phone call won't suffice). For example, we might arrange an impromptu meeting if we have a question about the validity of some aspect of a participating nurse's portfolio. Or we might meet if, during a mentoring session, a participating nurse asks a question, and we want to make sure we agree on how to respond to it. We also meet to prep for the presentation ceremony.

## *Offering Mentoring Support*

As members of the IMPACT committee, we offer mentoring support when needed to current and future participants. Mentoring sessions can be conducted one-on-one, via email, or by phone. During these sessions, we may:

- Provide guidance on successfully navigating the program

- Offer coaching on next steps as participants look to complete the activities required

- Introduce nurses to other mentors (such as clinical nurse specialists or nurse educators) to help them complete their IMPACT Program project

- Guide nurses to other programs in the organization (such as the Evidence-Based Practice [EBP] Fellowship program or the Research Fellowship program) to help them complete their IMPACT Program project

Basically, we're cheerleaders, rooting program participants on! This is truly one of the most enjoyable aspects of our job.

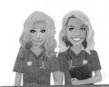

## MAKES SENSE

IMPACT participants are not required to meet with us, but we are available if they want the support.

To be clear, these mentoring sessions are meant to provide support and guidance *only*. They're not to ensure a prospective participant's acceptance into the IMPACT Program or to guarantee the approval of a current participant's portfolio. Taking this approach to mentoring enables us to maintain our objectivity (CHMC, 2016).

During our mentoring sessions, we have fielded questions ranging from "What are the program requirements?" to "What is a PowerPoint, and how do you create one?" This reflects the range of experience among nurses who have applied: from two years to 38 years. Some of our more experienced nurses have not written a paper or used a computer (except to chart a patient) in decades. But working with nurses on both ends of the spectrum has been so rewarding, whether it's a newer nurse who realizes she can make significant changes that have an enormous impact on patients across the enterprise or one with decades of experience who reignites his passion for nursing and his impact on the future of patient care.

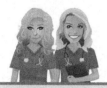

## PRICELESS

Mentoring not only greatly benefits our nurses, stimulating professional and personal growth, but also is instrumental to the success of the program as a whole.

## MELLISA

Not too long ago, a clinical nurse with three years of experience submitted a letter of intent to complete level 1 of the IMPACT Program. She asked if I could meet with her to talk through her project and activities.

When we met, she explained that she had completed an EBP project that was subsequently implemented in her area. However, she also revealed that the majority of her work for that project had been completed outside the 15-month time frame requirement—meaning she could not count it toward her IMPACT efforts. Needless to say, she was disappointed.

It occurred to me to ask her some questions about the implementation of her findings within her area—which, it turned out, *had* occurred within the 15-month time frame. She realized that by pivoting from an EBP project to a process improvement (PI) project, she could apply much of the work she'd already done toward the IMPACT Program. Fast-forward to the present: This nurse's project outcomes had such a positive impact on our organization, our CEO personally invited her to present her PI project at the next hospital board meeting.

# JUDY

Recently, a clinical nurse with more than 38 years of experience applied for the IMPACT Program. She wanted to advance professionally but had no desire to go back to school. She saw the IMPACT Program as a way to fill something she felt was missing in her professional career.

When I met with this nurse, I quickly realized that she had loads of great ideas for improving patient care. What she lacked was a way to move them forward. The IMPACT Program pushed her to do that—and when I say pushed her, I mean pushed her, as in way out of her comfort zone.

When she started the IMPACT Program, this nurse had no idea of what a PowerPoint was (let alone how to present information in narrative form), had never delivered a presentation in front of a group (not even her peers), and was terrified of trying anything new. But believe it or not, this nurse went on to complete the program not once, not twice, but *three times*. She is now a PowerPoint expert, has delivered multiple presentations organization-wide, and has led multiple EBPs with improved patient outcomes. And guess what: She is now getting ready to publish—yes, I said publish—her findings!

## *Reviewing Portfolios*

As program leaders, we review all portfolios, with each of us reviewing half of the portfolios submitted. The review process usually takes about four weeks. After we finish reviewing each portfolio, we scan it so we can keep an electronic copy on file.

When reviewing portfolios, we refer to a rubric that is identical to the explanation of activities document discussed in Chapter 5. We also use a portfolio planning form, also discussed in Chapter 5. This ensures a transparent, objective, and consistent approach for all applicants (CHMC, 2015).

Each portfolio takes about one to two hours to review. The process entails reading each section of the portfolio and referring to the rubric for each activity listed. If all criteria for an activity are met, we check off that activity on the portfolio planning form, indicating its acceptance (see Figures 8.1 and 8.2). If a nurse's portfolio meets all program requirements, the nurse transitions to the next phase of the IMPACT Program.

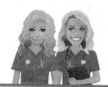

## MAKES SENSE

When assessing whether all criteria for an activity are met, we take an all-or-nothing approach. Either you met them all (in which case we count the activity) or you didn't (in which case we don't). We don't award partial credit.

**Portfolio Planning Form**
**Level 1**

Applicant Name/Credentials: **Mellisa Renter, BSN, RN, CPN**

Submission Date: **04/01/2021**

| | |
|---|:---:|
| **CLINICAL**<br>Three activities in at least two areas<br>(Must have an EBP, PI, or Research activity) | ☑ |
| 1. **PI: Infusion Center FTE Utilization Improvement** | ☑ |
| 2. **Policy/Procedure Development: Rituxan** | ☑ |
| 3. **Expanded Role: Auditor CLABSI Standardization** | ☑ |
| **EDUCATIONAL**<br>Three activities in at least two areas + at least 25 contact hours/year<br>(Must have an evidence-based inservice or podium presentation) | ☑ |
| Number of Contact Hours: **25** | ☑ |
| 1. **Podium Presentation: Infusion Center FTE Utilization** | ☑ |
| 2. **Enrichment Course: Hunters Syndrome Presentation** | ☑ |
| 3. **Enrichment Course: Xatemp Presentation** | ☑ |
| **PROFESSIONAL**<br>Three activities in at least two areas + Specialty Certification<br>(Volunteer and professional organization membership can only be used once) | ☑ |
| Specialty Certification: **CPN** | ☑ |
| 1. **Additional Certification: Chemotherapy and Biotherapy Provider** | ☑ |
| 2. **Professional Organization Membership: Association of Hematology Oncology Nurses – President** | ☑ |
| 3. **Professional Organization Membership: Association of Hematology Oncology Nurses – President** | ☑ |

**FIGURE 8.1** Portfolio planning form: Level 1.

**Portfolio Planning Form**
**Level 2**

**Name/Credentials: Judy Thomas, BSN, RN, CCRN, CPN**

**Submission Date: 04/01/2021**

| | |
|---|:---:|
| **CLINICAL**<br>Must have an EBP, PI, or Research activity that impacts across the continuum of care<br>(Another area has been educated on the topic for potential/actual implementation) | ☑ |
| 1. <u>**EBP Project: Nurse-Driven Foley Removal Algorithm**</u> | ☑ |
| **EDUCATIONAL**<br>Four activities in at least three areas + at least 31 contact hours/year<br>(Must have an activity where you educated beyond your area a change in practice in which<br>you played a key role in dissemination of knowledge) | ☑ |
| Number of Contact Hours: **32.75** | ☑ |
| 1. <u>**EBP Presentation: Nurse-Driven Foley Removal Algorithm to PICU Staff**</u> | ☑ |
| 2. <u>**EBP Presentation: Nurse-Driven Foley Removal Algorithm to Five Med-Surg Staff**</u> | ☑ |
| 3. <u>**Healthcare Academic Course: Nursing 722 Childcare Management**</u> | ☑ |
| 4. <u>**Enrichment Course: Pediatric Surgical Service Conference**</u> | ☑ |
| **PROFESSIONAL**<br>Four activities in at least three areas + Specialty Certification<br>(Volunteer and professional organization membership can only be used once) | ☑ |
| Specialty Certification: **CPN** | ☑ |
| 1. <u>**Additional Certification: CCRN**</u> | ☑ |
| 2. <u>**Committee Council: PICU HAC Committee**</u> | ☑ |
| 3. <u>**Professional Organization Membership: AACN**</u> | ☑ |
| 4. <u>**Community Volunteer: ENOA Meals on Wheels**</u> | ☑ |

**FIGURE 8.2** Portfolio planning form: Level 2.

## Dealing With Missing Portfolio Components

Now, this is rare, but it has happened: One of us goes to review a portfolio, only to discover that it is missing some required component. When this happens, the program leader who initially reviewed the portfolio hands it off to the other program leader for a second review. The second reviewer then reviews only the section in question. This is to ensure the first reviewer hasn't just missed something (CHMC, 2016).

If, after the second review is finished, we agree that the required component is indeed missing, one of two things happens (CHMC, 2016):

- If the nurse submitted for level 2, we determine whether she has met the requirements for level 1. If so, we send the nurse a letter that identifies what is missing from the portfolio. The letter also offers the nurse the opportunity to proceed as a level 1 participant or to discuss how to resubmit her portfolio for the next review period as a level 2 participant.

- If the nurse failed to meet the requirements for level 1 or level 2, we send the nurse a letter that identifies what is missing from the portfolio, informs the nurse that he will not advance to the next phase of the IMPACT Model, and invites him to a mentoring session to discuss next steps for resubmitting his portfolio for the next review period (see Figure 8.3).

[NAME],

Thank you for your interest in the IMPACT Reward and Recognition Program at Children's Hospital & Medical Center. During the review of your portfolio, there were key items missing, which prevents you from moving on to the presentation phase of the program.

We encourage you to continue working on your portfolio and activities for future submissions. Please contact Mellisa Renter, Director of Professional Nursing Practice, by email (mrenter@childrensomaha.org) or by phone (402-955-4180) if you would like to schedule a time to review your portfolio for future submissions.

Sincerely,

The IMPACT Review Committee

**Items Missing:**

- Level 2 Performance Improvement Project
  - o Outcomes of the project to prove <u>sustainment</u>
    - ▪ Must show three post-data points on at least two metrics/goals
  - o Team Charter

- Presentation within CHMC
  - o No supporting evidence submitted

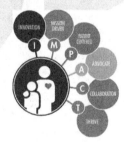

8200 Dodge Street  |  Omaha, NE 68114-4113  |  402-955-5400  |  ChildrensOmaha.org

**FIGURE 8.3** Participant letter—missing components.

We do not allow participants to resubmit their portfolio for the same review period. They must wait until the next review period—no exceptions (CHMC, 2015). In the intervening period, we offer to work with participants to help them get their portfolio where it needs to be. Some participants need only minimal guidance; others need lots of

*Continued*

**Dealing With Missing Portfolio Components**
*Continued*

help. That's OK! The important thing is that they stick with it for their own professional growth.

Note that all activities in the resubmitted portfolio must fall within the new 15-month time frame. If an activity falls out of that time frame, the participant must complete a different activity to replace it (CHMC, 2015).

## *Handling Appeals*

Participants whose portfolios do not meet program requirements and who do not move on to the last phase of the program can submit an appeal form (see Figure 8.4). They have 14 days to do so.

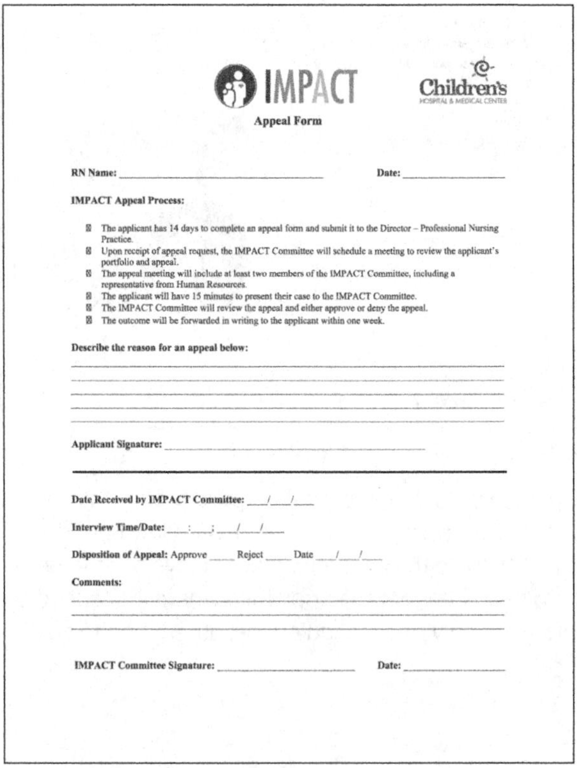

IMPACT Children's HOSPITAL & MEDICAL CENTER

**Appeal Form**

**RN Name:** ____________________ **Date:** __________

**IMPACT Appeal Process:**

- The applicant has 14 days to complete an appeal form and submit it to the Director – Professional Nursing Practice.
- Upon receipt of appeal request, the IMPACT Committee will schedule a meeting to review the applicant's portfolio and appeal.
- The appeal meeting will include at least two members of the IMPACT Committee, including a representative from Human Resources.
- The applicant will have 15 minutes to present their case to the IMPACT Committee.
- The IMPACT Committee will review the appeal and either approve or deny the appeal.
- The outcome will be forwarded in writing to the applicant within one week.

**Describe the reason for an appeal below:**

**Applicant Signature:** ____________________

**Date Received by IMPACT Committee:** ___/___/___

**Interview Time/Date:** ___:___; ___/___/___

**Disposition of Appeal:** Approve ____ Reject ____ Date ___/___/___

**Comments:**

**IMPACT Committee Signature:** ____________________ **Date:** __________

**FIGURE 8.4** IMPACT appeal form.

When a participant submits an appeal form, a second review will occur that includes at least two members of the IMPACT committee (CNO will be one of them), including the SVP of HR. The committee of the two members plus the HR representative then schedules a meeting with the participant to review the appeal. During this meeting, the participant has 15 minutes to present his or her case. Afterward, the committee reviews the appeal as a group and either approves it or denies it. The outcome of the appeal is sent to the participant in writing within one week (CHMC, 2015).

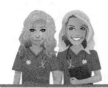

## CHECK

At Children's, we have never had a participant submit an appeal. This is because the program is so objective, there is little to no room to argue when a portfolio is rejected. Still, it's important to have a clear appeal process in place.

## *Planning the Presentation Ceremony*

As mentioned in Chapter 7, after the completion of the review process, the IMPACT committee sends a letter to all nurses who qualify for phase 3 of the IMPACT Program. This letter congratulates the nurses and invites them to a ceremony to present their portfolio (CHMC, 2016). We also send invitations to the presentation ceremony by email to our organization's CEO, CNO, CMO, SVP of HR, nurse directors, nurse managers, clinical nurse specialists, nurse educators, clinical nurses, providers, and other nurses throughout the organization. We hold these presentation ceremonies twice a year—once for each review period— and we look forward to them every single time.

As you learned in Chapter 7, each ceremony starts with a welcome and introduction address, delivered by the program leaders (us). During this address, we introduce ourselves, offer a quick overview of the program's purpose, discuss its impact on clinical nurse retention to date, and touch on various projects completed by participating nurses (including projects that were used to gain designations and redesignations). This is an important part to the ceremony because it reminds the executive team of the impact our program has on our organization's strategic initiatives. It also inspires other clinical nurses in attendance to consider participating in the program. After that, participating nurses deliver their PowerPoint presentations. Finally, we conduct the award ceremony and deliver final remarks. Figure 8.5 shows the agenda for a recent presentation ceremony at Children's.

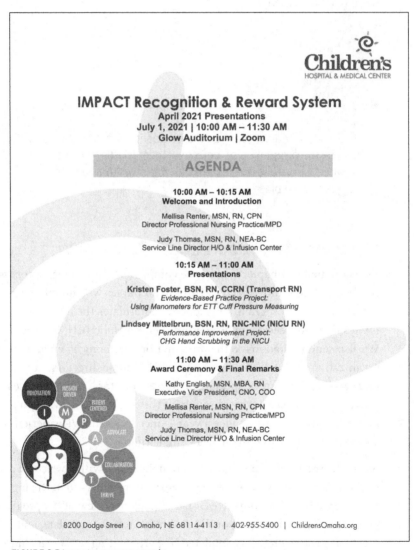

**FIGURE 8.5** Impact ceremony agenda.

## *Dealing With Compensation*

As program leaders, it's our job to email each program participant's manager at the end of each quarter to verify that the participant has met all eligibility requirements for compensation—in other words, that the person successfully completed the IMPACT Program and has continued to serve as a clinical nurse. If nurses don't meet both these eligibility requirements—for example, if they are promoted to a supervisory role—then their quarterly compensation will be prorated accordingly. Once we verify that eligibility requirements have been met, we send an email to HR to approve payment (CHMC, 2016).

# *MORE ON SUSTAINABILITY*

To enable two program leaders who have other full-time responsibilities to sustain the IMPACT Program (with the assistance of the rest of the IMPACT committee), we needed to design the program to consume few resources and minimal time. To achieve this, we intentionally designed the program to place the bulk of the work on participating nurses, with minimal leadership oversight. To that end, we developed the following tools and policies (CHMC, 2015):

- **Limited portfolio submissions:** Rather than allowing nurses to submit portfolios anytime, we opted to accept portfolio submissions only twice per year (on April 1 and October 1). This allows us enough time to review one round of portfolios before the next round is submitted and to manage other aspects of the program, which in turn makes it easier to facilitate and sustain the program.

- **Educational PowerPoint presentation:** To educate nurses about the IMPACT Model, we developed an educational PowerPoint presentation. Nurses who are interested in participating in the program must review this presentation in its entirety. If a participating nurse comes to either of us with a question that is answered in the PowerPoint presentation, we direct the nurse to that resource.

- **Policy document:** All components of the IMPACT Model are spelled out in a detailed policy document. This is to ensure that all applicants and participants have a clear understanding of program requirements. Nurses with questions about a particular policy item are directed to this document.

- **Letter of intent form:** Requiring nurses who are interested in participating in the IMPACT Program to complete a letter of intent form gives us some idea of how many portfolios we can expect for the next review period. This enables us to plan our calendars accordingly. The letter of intent form also helps us ensure that applicants meet the initial requirements to apply.

- **Explanation of activities document and activity forms:** These were instrumental in minimizing the need for extensive leadership oversight. The explanation of activities document outlines everything required for portfolio narratives and spells out which activity forms must be signed and turned in. We created separate forms for each activity so we wouldn't have to verify the validity of everything written in the narrative. We require specific key stakeholders to sign these forms to ensure that the contents of the narratives are accurate.

- **Presentation template:** We send each participant who advances to phase 3 a PowerPoint presentation template, which they use to generate their portfolio presentations. This template helps participants ensure all components are covered without requiring significant guidance from members of the IMPACT committee.

- **Portfolio planning form:** This form is required and acts as a guide to participants as well as a checklist for us as we review the portfolios once sent in. This form is helpful for participating nurses because it acts as an overall road map of what they need to include in their portfolio and ensures they have checked off required elements. (Refer to Figures 8.1 and 8.2.)

- **Review rubric:** The review rubric is identical to the explanation of activities document used by program participants. It supports an objective, methodical, streamlined, and efficient portfolio-review process, which saves time and effort.

One more thing: As program leaders, we have full authority to implement any enhancements needed with little to no red tape. Indeed, the only time we need to clear changes with the CNO or the SVP of HR is if they involve a financial investment.

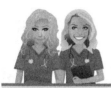

## SMART!

Developing tools to enable participating nurses to complete the IMPACT Program more or less autonomously does more than support sustainability. It also represents an opportunity for professional development among participating nurses.

# REFERENCES

Children's Hospital & Medical Center. (2015). *Children's Hospital & Medical Center.* Omaha, Nebraska.

Children's Hospital & Medical Center. (2016). *Children's Hospital & Medical Center.* Omaha, Nebraska.

> *"Leadership is not about control but service. It is not about power but empowerment."*
>
> —Myles Munroe

## CHAPTER 9

# Getting Organizational Buy-In

## INTRODUCTION

Normally, when an individual leader or group of leaders proposes big changes to an organization—especially ones that involve a significant financial investment—people can *freak out!* So, you're probably wondering how in the world we were able to persuade our leaders and our nurses to buy into a big change initiative like the IMPACT Model—let alone continue to support it over the years. Great question! This chapter will answer it.

## OBTAINING BUY-IN AMONG KEY LEADERS

One person's desired outcome from a proposed change might be totally different from another's. For example, clinical leaders may like a proposed program because it promotes more autonomy and satisfaction among nurses, while organizational leaders might be keen on it because it improves patient outcomes—or, in this case, nurse retention. So, before we did anything else, including forming the IMPACT committee, we needed to identify the desired outcomes for various groups so we could design a program that satisfied everyone.

First, we focused on our CNO and SVP of HR. Before we even set up our initial meeting with these two key stakeholders, we gathered some revealing statistics to support the need for a new model to improve clinical nurse retention:

- The average turnover rate of RNs at hospitals nationwide was 17.8% (NSI Nursing Solutions, 2020).

- The average cost per nurse of each instance of turnover was between $33,300 and $56,000 (NSI Nursing Solutions, 2020). Hospitals lose on average between $5.2 million and $8.0 million annually due to bedside nurse turnover (Vaughn, 2020).

- Clinical nurse turnover at Children's Hospital was 9.9% and increasing.

- Only 86.06% of clinical nurses at Children's Hospital responded "yes" to a survey question asking whether they planned to stay on their unit.

- Experts predict a nursing shortage by 2025 as more baby boomers retire (American Association of Colleges of Nursing, 2020).

- Our local nursing schools offered limited pediatric education, resulting in fewer new nurses entering that specialty area.

- Children's Hospital was building a new facility, the Hubbard Center for Children, whose completion would result in an increased need for clinical nurses amidst a nurse shortage in the area (Children's Hospital & Medical Center [CHMC], 2015).

Our clinical leaders cared about all these issues, but addressing them was not their highest priority. So, before meeting with *that* key stakeholder group, we brainstormed what outcomes of a nurse-retention model they might find beneficial, based on information they had provided us in the past. We came up with the following:

- Increased clinical nurse autonomy

- Improved patient outcomes

- Improved patient satisfaction

- More engaged clinical nurses

- Improved clinical nurse satisfaction

- Improved retention

- Easier recruiting

- Improved work-life balance

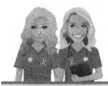

## LET'S DISCUSS

It was really important to us to obtain buy-in from clinical nurse leaders and to involve them in the early stages of model planning because we wanted the program to benefit those closest to the work. This doesn't always happen when programs are driven by organizational leaders.

Armed with all this information, we met with members of both groups to increase awareness of the issue of nurse retention and inspire in them a desire to drive change alongside us. And, well, it worked! Ultimately, the IMPACT Model was developed and approved by our CNO, the SVP of HR, and nursing leadership, at which point our CNO added it to the nursing executive budget (CHMC, 2015). In addition, our CNO, SVP of HR, and some nurse leaders served on the original IMPACT committee. This helped legitimize the program and sustain its momentum.

Some of you may be wondering, doesn't all this upfront work take longer? Our answer is this: Working upfront to lock in support from the very first meeting takes less time than failing to win over key stakeholders and being sent back to the drawing board. It also increases the likelihood that you will successfully convince key stakeholders to sign on sooner rather than later. This is critical because if you're shot down the first time you present your idea, it'll be much harder to get buy-in the second time around.

# *GAINING BROADER ORGANIZATIONAL BUY-IN*

Initial support for the IMPACT Model from our CNO, SVP of HR, and clinical leaders was enough to roll it out. But to sustain it, we would eventually need additional buy-in—specifically, CEO, COO, and executive director of finance. This happened about two years after the program started.

Convincing this group to offer ongoing support for a program is never easy. This is especially true when there's a price tag involved and when, because the program is relatively new, there's little in the way of outcomes to prove its worth. So, we developed an executive summary, which our CNO and SVP of HR presented to the executives in question. The executive summary included the following sections:

- **Background:** This contained the statistical information we had shared with the CNO, SVP of HR, and clinical leaders. It also included information about why clinical nurses were leaving the bedside and the impact of this trend on patient outcomes and organizational strategic initiatives. Finally, it noted that the program is essentially a reward and recognition system to encourage nurses to stay at the bedside—which strategically aligned with Children's mission, vision, and strategic initiatives.

- **IMPACT Model details and highlights:** This contained the IMPACT Model purpose statement and discussed key program components.

- **Outcomes:** This focused on clinical outcomes, showcasing various projects and how they aligned with organizational strategic initiatives. It also covered the average cost of the program per fiscal year compared to funds saved due to a resulting decrease in RN turnover. (Chapter 10 discusses IMPACT Program outcomes in more detail.)

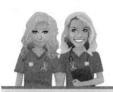

## PRICELESS

Having a passionate and committed CNO and SVP of HR was invaluable in gaining initial buy-in for the IMPACT Model. But once the program got going, it was its outcomes and results that drove ongoing support.

We also leveraged the presentation ceremony, which occurs in phase 3 of the IMPACT Program, to ensure continued organizational buy-in and support. We even timed the first of these ceremonies with our delivery of the executive summary to remind the executive team of program outcomes and benefits. Attending the presentation ceremony enabled members of this team to see the passion and drive behind the program firsthand.

Inviting our executive team to presentation ceremonies has done wonders to sustain the IMPACT Program. Twice a year, the executive team is reminded how the program has contributed to strategic initiatives. The ceremony also provides them with an opportunity to engage directly with participating nurses. Indeed, it has renewed the executive team's appreciation of our clinical nurses' knowledge and expertise, which helps them—and all of us—meet our mission, "to improve the life of every child through dedication to exceptional clinical care, advocacy research, and education," and our vision, "to be the global leader for children's health."

# PERSUADING NURSES TO JOIN THE IMPACT PROGRAM

Many of our nurse leaders, including our supervisors, nurse educators, clinical nurse specialists, department directors, and even providers, are strong advocates of the IMPACT Model. This is important for lots of reasons—not least of which is that they can encourage nurses to participate in the program. When our nurse leaders encounter nurses who want to grow within the profession but remain at the bedside, they guide them to the IMPACT Program. They also help mentor nurses who decide to participate in the program, connecting them to key stakeholders and other resources to ensure they succeed.

IMPACT Program participants also advocate for the program, recruiting many of their peers to apply and mentoring them throughout the program. Recently, a clinical nurse who worked on our emergency transport team completed the IMPACT Program. During the review process, she mentioned conversations she'd had with some of her peers about the program. She went on to say that she was encouraging these peers to apply, as they were already engaged in several activities that would count toward activity points. Her encouragement acted as an informal way of recruitment for the program.

# REFERENCES

American Association of Colleges of Nursing. (2020, September). *Nursing shortage.* https://www.aacnnursing.org/News-Information/Fact-Sheets/Nursing-Shortage

Children's Hospital & Medical Center. (2015). *Children's Hospital & Medical Center.* Omaha, Nebraska.

NSI Nursing Solutions. (2020). *2020 NSI National Health Care Retention & RN Staffing Report.* https://www.nsinursingsolutions.com/Documents/Library/NSI_National_Health_Care_Retention_Report.pdf

Vaughn, N. (2020, October 27). *Nurse turnover rates: How to reduce healthcare turnover.* https://www.relias.com/blog/how-to-reduce-healthcare-turnover

## CHAPTER 10

# IMPACT Model and Project Outcomes

## INTRODUCTION

When we launched the IMPACT Model, we honestly had no idea how impactful it would be. Sometimes we pinch ourselves to remember that we created an amazing clinical nurse retention program that has proven to be so much more than what we imagined!

The impact of the program is perhaps best illustrated by various projects completed by participating nurses that have gone on to influence our organization's mission, vision, strategic plan, and patient outcomes. This chapter discusses several of these projects in the following areas:

- Operational excellence

- Nurse autonomy and advocacy

- Interprofessional collaboration and cross-continuum alignment

- Wise use of resources

- Improved patient outcomes

This chapter also discusses key outcomes of the IMPACT Program as a whole.

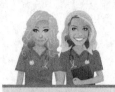

## SQUAD

So many clinical nurses think they can't make a difference—that they're "just" clinical nurses. Well, knock that off! Clinical nurses have a frontline view of healthcare and what needs changing. Our job as leaders is to listen to clinical nurses so we can shape the future of healthcare *together*.

# OPERATIONAL EXCELLENCE PI PROJECT: FTE UTILIZATION IMPROVEMENT IN THE INFUSION CENTER

A registered nurse with six years of experience who had worked for two years in our infusion center noticed that the center wasn't running as efficiently as it could be, which resulted in dissatisfaction among staff and patients. She designed her IMPACT Program project to tackle this problem by addressing how the staffing pattern and hours of operation were occurring in the infusion center. Specifically, she wanted to find ways to address the following goals:

- Reduce unpaid hours when drops in census led to staff not getting paid for their full FTE, due to either not having enough PTO (personal time off) to cover or a desire to save these hours for a planned vacation

- Improve work/life balance for staff members, while also ensuring that the needs of all patients were met

The nurse determined that she could achieve these goals by taking two critical steps:

- Extending the infusion center's hours of operation to include evening and weekend appointments

- Streamlining the appointment-scheduling process

Project outcomes were as follows:

- Extended hours of operation enabled parents to miss less work and children to miss less school, leading to increased patient satisfaction.

- Extended hours of operation resulted in a 75% improvement in staff achieving their actual FTE, without needing to use PTO, within the first six months of instituting the above critical steps.

- The number of processes needed to schedule patients dropped from 12 to 3, resulting in improved efficiency.

Ultimately, enabling patients to schedule appointments quickly and efficiently and at more convenient times had a global impact on the entire specialty pediatric clinic setting.

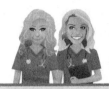

## UMMMM...

As a nurse leader, you might have freaked out a tiny bit when you saw that this project involved changing hours of operation. As leaders we struggle at times to think the staff may have some great thoughts/ideas on how the operations of an area can work—as we think, "That is *our* job"—and it can touch up our ego a little. But it is important to *lead* our staff and not *manage* them. So it's critical that you not declare any type of project off limits. Don't take anything off the table! When you allow yourself to lead your employees to think differently, it is amazing what they can achieve.

# NURSE AUTONOMY AND ADVOCACY EBP PROJECT: EMERGENT DELIRIUM IN THE PEDIATRIC SURGICAL PATIENT (PHASE 1 RECOVERY)

A registered nurse with 38 years of experience recognized that our organization did not have an accurate means of identifying emergence delirium in phase 1 recovery post-operative patients. Our post anesthesia care unit (PACU) nurses used the Face, Legs, Activity, Cry, Consolability pain scale along with subjective observation to assess and care for agitated phase 1 recovery patients. But because there was no clear way to identify emergence delirium, agitated patients received inconsistent treatment.

For her IMPACT Program project, this nurse worked with the anesthesia group to advocate on the patients' behalf in developing an evidence-based nurse-driven protocol to identify emergence delirium in the phase 1 recovery period. Nurse-driven protocols provide an autonomous practice, where nurses can use objective data to make decisions based on their scope of nursing practice without contacting a provider for orders. Project outcomes were as follows:

- Patient injuries (for example, due to the loss of IVs and drains) decreased.
- PACU wait times decreased.
- Parent satisfaction increased.

This protocol has since been expanded to other areas within the organization.

The nurse also partnered with another clinical nurse in the MRI department to conduct a research study that looks into emergence delirium in pediatric patients undergoing MRIs—a great example of how one project can lead to another!

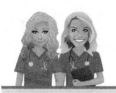

## CHECK

> IMPACT Program projects help us reach our organizational strategic initiatives and provide the best care for our patients.

# INTERPROFESSIONAL COLLABORATION AND CROSS-CONTINUUM ALIGNMENT EBP PROJECT: PREVENTING NULYTELY ASPIRATION

A registered nurse with two years of experience observed that there were no policies or guidelines, standardized dosing, assessment, monitoring, or ordering processes for the administration of NuLytely to patients. She developed her IMPACT Program project to address this.

With mentoring and guidance from multiple individuals, this nurse led a group consisting of nurses from her area, a clinical nurse specialist, five medical directors across the continuum of care, and members of our performance improvement and nursing education staff to create a policy and order set to guide the care of patients on NuLytely. Project outcomes were as follows:

- A policy and procedure were put in place to guide nursing care.
- An order set was put in place to guide ordering and administration.
- Zero aspirations occurred within the first six months of implementation, ultimately leading to decreased pain and significant health risk to the patients.

Simply put, this young nurse saw an opportunity to improve patient care within her own area and quickly realized that the outcomes could—and did—affect care throughout the organization. She has now set a goal to publish the guidelines and outcomes for further dissemination.

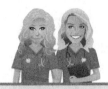

## *MAKES SENSE*

Interprofessional collaboration and cross-continuum alignment are so important for a nurse's professional development. Too often, projects are done in isolation, preventing other areas from improving processes and care. This is why having a cross-continuum influence is a level 2 requirement of the IMPACT Model.

# *WISE USE OF RESOURCES PI PROJECT: CHG HAND SCRUBBING IN THE NICU*

A nurse with three years of experience observed that a two-minute hand scrub with chlorhexidine gluconate (CHG) was required at the start of each shift in the neonatal intensive care unit (NICU). This practice had been in place for quite some time.

In studying the issue, the nurse discovered that there was little evidence to support this practice. The nurse also observed that with all the tasks required at the start of a shift—such as obtaining reports from the off-going nurse, attending to family and patient needs, logging on to computers and phones, and looking over orders, labs, and notes—there was a high risk of interruption during the two-minute hand scrub.

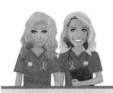

## UMMMM...

When someone answers, "We've always done it that way" when asked about a process or practice, it almost always means it could be improved!

For her IMPACT Program project, this nurse decided to create a hand-washing protocol based on current evidence to protect the vulnerable NICU population from unwanted pathogens while maximizing nurse efficiency. This protocol called for the discontinuation of the two-minute CHG hand scrub at the start of each shift; instead, nurses should use alcohol-based hand sanitizer or, if their hands were visibly soiled, soap and water on a routine basis throughout their shift. The project outcomes were as follows:

- The organization saved $13,485.89 in the first year by decreasing the use of CHG hand scrub.

- On average, the organization saves 340 clinical nurse hours each year.

- 60% of nurses reported greater efficiency.

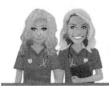

## PRICELESS

The IMPACT Model challenges clinical nurses to make a difference not only in patient care but also to the organization's financial success.

# IMPROVED PATIENT OUTCOMES EBP PROJECT: NURSE-DRIVEN FOLEY REMOVAL ALGORITHM

A nurse with five years of experience observed that the PICU had a high number of Foley catheter days and no standardized algorithm for Foley removal. She decided to develop a nurse-driven Foley removal algorithm and protocol for use in her area and for submission as her IMPACT Program project. This required support from nursing leadership, providers, and performance improvement staff, as well as multiple committees. The project outcomes were as follows:

- Within two months of implementation, the PICU experienced a 40% reduction in Foley catheter days.

- The PICU had zero catheter-associated urinary infections for more than a year.

Nurse-driven protocols facilitate autonomy and empower nurses to practice at the height of their abilities. They also help improve efficiency in patient care, enabling nurses to provide timely care without the need to call a provider.

# PROGRAM OUTCOMES

Our main goal with the IMPACT Model was to improve our clinical nurse retention rate. Well, we are elated to report that the IMPACT Model did just that! The year the program launched, our clinical nurse turnover rate was 9.90%. The next year, the rate declined to 9.53%. The year after that, it dropped to 8.86%. In addition:

- In the four years since the IMPACT Program launched, 97% of program participants still work at the bedside, and 2.5% have moved into a leadership role within the organization.

- During the same period, clinical nurses within the organization reported a job enjoyment rate ranging from 4.48 to 4.55—much higher than the national mean range of 4.17 to 4.23 (National Database of Nursing Quality Indicators [NDNQI], 2018). As you know, when staff enjoy their work, they are more apt to stay.

- The percentage of clinical nurses at Children's planning to stay on in their same unit rose from 86.06% to 90.06% within two years. This reflects the influence of IMPACT Program participants on their peers.

In addition to improving clinical nurse retention, the IMPACT Program has had a positive influence in the following areas:

- The mean range of ratings for the professional status of nurses within our organization is 4.69 to 4.79 (compared to a national mean range of 4.43 to 4.52; NDNQI, 2018).

- The mean range of ratings of strong interprofessional relationships within our organization is 4.09 to 4.18 (NDNQI, 2018). This can be attributed in part to the networking and collaborating done by IMPACT Program participants with non-nurse stakeholders as they complete program activities.

- The mean range of RN to MD interaction ratings within our organization is 4.82 to 4.92 (compared to a national mean range of 4.58 to 4.62; NDNQI, 2018). IMPACT Program participants collaborating with physicians as they complete program activities has helped positively influence this measure.

- 84% of nurses within our organization (including all IMPACT Program participants) hold professional certifications.

- 80% of IMPACT Program participants have become members of professional organizations.

Finally, the IMPACT Model has improved organizational outcomes, cross-continuum patient care, and patient satisfaction; promoted shared decision-making; driven succession planning, professional development, and community support through volunteering; cultivated a positive culture; increased nursing knowledge within our walls; and more.

# REFERENCE

National Database of Nursing Quality Indicators. (2018). National Database of Nursing Quality Indicators.

*"It is a beautiful thing when a career and a passion come together."*

—Unknown

## CHAPTER 11

# Professional Journey: Clinical Nurse

## INTRODUCTION

Think how you would feel about an organization that empowers, recognizes, and invests in you. Wouldn't you be more apt to remain there? That's the idea behind the IMPACT Model: to empower, recognize, and invest in nurses who make an impact on the organization's mission, vision, and strategic initiatives. It's no wonder, then, that the IMPACT Model has not only yielded impressive project and program outcomes but has also had a profound effect on the professional journey of participating nurses. That's what this chapter is about.

## NURSE EMPOWERMENT → NURSE ENGAGEMENT → NURSE RETENTION

Way back in this book's introduction, we discussed how a lack of empowerment created a negative cascading effect that ultimately resulted in low nurse retention. Actively empowering nurses in your organization can be a game changer. Among other positive outcomes, nurse empowerment can lead to (George et al., 2002):

- Increased work satisfaction

- Better patient outcomes

- Increased nurse autonomy

Who *wouldn't* want to work with motivated nurses who not only identify opportunities for improvement but also innovate solutions and roll up their sleeves to implement them?

Empowerment drives engagement, and through engagement comes retention. As leaders we need to grab ahold of those voicing their thoughts on improvement opportunities and actively engage in mentoring and developing them toward creating the outcomes necessary for organizations to thrive into the future. When leaders take a step back and empower those closest to the work, they positively affect how nurses perceive their workplace environment, ultimately leading to retention (DiNapoli et al., 2016).

Simply put, the purpose of the IMPACT Model is to empower and engage nurses to drive nurse retention and other positive organizational outcomes (see Figure 11.1).

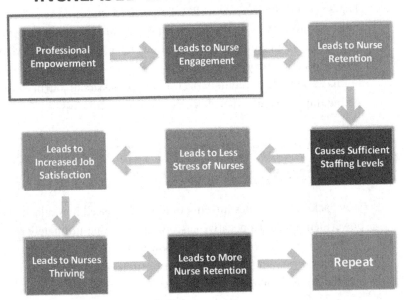

**FIGURE 11.1** Increased empowerment effect.

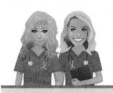

## PRICELESS

Nurses who participate in the IMPACT Program enjoy significant empowerment, autonomy, and professional development. The outcome: engagement, retention, and a career as a frontline clinical nurse.

# *PERSONAL IMPACT*

The IMPACT Model produces wonderful organizational outcomes. But perhaps the most exceptional program outcome is the professional development and growth of participating nurses. With the IMPACT Model, the nurse's journey is the priority, not just the activities and outcomes.

Professional development of the clinical nurse is a key element of the IMPACT Program journey, helping to drive nurse empowerment and engagement. Opportunities for professional development within the program include the following:

- **Completing an evidence-based practice, process improvement, or research project:** These projects enable participating nurses to partner with peers and leaders and to develop the skills needed to complete other high-caliber projects.

- **Presenting in front of peers and leaders:** The IMPACT Program affords participating nurses several opportunities to build this skill. For example, all participating nurses are required to present their portfolio and outcomes during phase 3 of the program. In addition, they can present their project to earn activity points in the educational category.

- **Sharpening communication skills:** With multiple activities needed to accomplish the program, the participating nurse must reach out to a multitude of individuals and engage in conversations. This is definitely a growth opportunity as they learn about networking and how to change their communication style depending on the target audience.

- **Instilling confidence to question norms:** Empowering nurses to question why we do things the way we do is invaluable. A quality, safety, and best practice mindset influences how nurses think through their everyday practice and furthers professional development.

These are just a few examples of professional development opportunities offered by the IMPACT Model. Others will vary depending on what activities participating nurses choose to complete the program. Every nurse's journey is unique.

The impact of these professional development opportunities may differ depending on the nurse's experience. What may be considered a small-scale professional achievement for a more experienced nurse could be a huge achievement for another nurse who is newer to practice. Again, this is unique to each individual nurse.

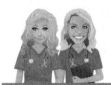 *CHECK*

Giving nurses the autonomy to choose the activities they participate in also plays a part in their professional development journey.

As mentioned, during phase 3, IMPACT Program participants present their portfolio in front of peers and organizational leaders. Afterward, some of these participants may be invited to present in front of other forums. These can include the following:

- **The transformational report out:** The purpose of this quarterly organizational forum is to share and celebrate projects and outcomes from across the continuum that have positively influenced the organization's mission, vision, and strategic initiatives. Most presenters in this forum are managers, directors, and vice presidents, so when a clinical nurse is invited to present, it is an incredible honor. It's also an incredible professional development opportunity—made even better by forum leaders, who mentor nurses who are invited to present to prepare them for the event. Several IMPACT Program participants have presented at this forum, with great success.

- **The hospital board meeting:** After hearing a nurse's phase 3 IMPACT Program portfolio presentation, our CEO may personally invite the nurse to present at the next board meeting—another incredible honor. In this case, the participating nurse's director typically assists in developing a PowerPoint presentation geared toward board members. Again, several IMPACT Program participants have successfully presented at this forum.

That's not all. Some IMPACT Program participants—urged on by key stakeholders—have shared their projects and outcomes on a regional or even national level. For example, several program participants have published their findings in prestigious journals. Others have delivered presentations at conferences. Several expert leaders within our organization serve as mentors to guide participating nurses through these processes, which is an amazing investment in our clinical staff. Again, this is a huge compliment to the participating nurse. It also urges the nurse to think beyond his department, and even beyond the organization as a whole.

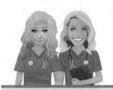

## GOOD IDEA

As an organization, we make every effort to enable our nursing staff to deliver poster or podium presentations at conferences. This gives our nurses the opportunity to develop professionally while also promoting the organization on a regional or national level. But sometimes we just don't have the budget for it. In that case, we may urge interested nurses to apply discretionary funds from their IMPACT Program compensation package to that end. These discretionary funds are discussed in Chapter 7.

One great outcome that we didn't anticipate is that after nurses complete the IMPACT Program, they often continue to drive positive changes within the organization. Sometimes they do this by becoming actively involved in other projects. Other times it's by assuming an expanded role. Or they may even decide to participate in the IMPACT Program again—for example, to achieve level 2 status after completing level 1.

We've also seen IMPACT Program participants advocate for, empower, and influence their peers—encouraging others to think differently, get involved, and take an active approach to their role as a clinical nurse. Simply put, the IMPACT Program opens the eyes of participating nurses, enabling them to better understand our strategic initiatives and to connect the dots on how they can help meet them.

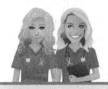

## MAKES SENSE

Having a system and culture that supports professional development is foundational to the success of the IMPACT Program and the clinical nurses who participate in it.

# *VOICES OF CLINICAL NURSES*

The program offers amazing opportunities to participants. But don't just take our word for it. Here are comments from several nurses who have completed all three phases:

*"Being part of IMPACT has pushed me to grow profession-ally and has encouraged me to learn new things. I had be-come complacent in my job after being here for 32 years, and now I have more to work for and look for opportunities to be more involved."*

*"Gained confidence in my ability to expand beyond my role as a nurse and advocate for other nurses. Able to live up to my personal career goal of feeling I make a difference in the lives of others. IMPACT gives nurses more autonomy to make changes and positively impact our organization."*

*"The program provides a way to recognize the nursing staff for the extra work they do to improve the lives of those we serve and those around us. It has pushed me out of my comfort zone by trying things in areas I would not have."*

*"I applied for the IMPACT Program because I wanted an opportunity to grow professionally as a bedside nurse without having to make the financial commitment of going back to school. The IMPACT Program has allowed me to make meaningful change in my unit through my perfor-mance improvement project, become a certified nurse in my specialty area, and volunteer my time to our hospital and community. This program gave me the opportunity to be more than just a bedside nurse and allowed me to see that change and quality improvement can happen at any professional level. Beyond that, this program helps to ensure the future financial success of my family. The IMPACT Program is what sets Children's apart and challenges us to continue to be our best for children that we serve."*

*Continued*

# VOICES OF CLINICAL NURSES (Continued)

*"If someone would have told me when I graduated nursing school that I would do a research project, write a policy and order set, and implement a change organization-wide at Children's in less than two years as a nurse, I would have never believed them. The reward of knowing I helped impact the safety of our patients through my participation in the IMPACT Program has been something indescribable."*

*"The work of our bedside nurses matters. Clinical nurses are the sharp edge of seeing what issues we face; when we're given the support and encouragement to solve these issues, we improve patient care."*

# THE IMPACT PROGRAM AND MASLOW'S HIERARCHY OF NEEDS

You've probably heard of Maslow's Hierarchy of Needs (Maslow, 1943). It describes a series of human needs that must be fulfilled for someone to achieve full development: physical survival, safety, belonging, esteem or importance, and self-actualization.

Interestingly, as shown in Figure 11.2, you can match up these needs with the needs for employee engagement. You can also see how the IMPACT Model addresses each one. Specifically:

- **Survival and security:** These levels are addressed by the compensation package awarded to IMPACT Program participants.

- **Belonging, importance, and self-actualization:** The IMPACT Model addresses these by communicating to nurses that the organization genuinely cares about them and their professional growth, by conveying that their opinions and contributions matter, by giving them the opportunity to learn and grow, and by empowering them to achieve.

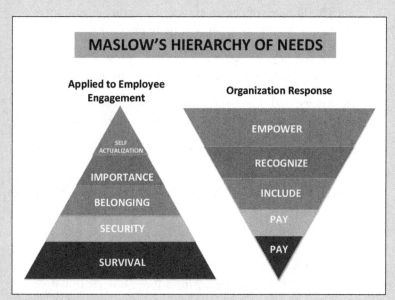

**FIGURE 11.2** Employee engagement hierarchy of needs.

Why does the IMPACT Model seek to meet these needs? Simple. Because nurses who reach the top of the hierarchy are engaged—and are therefore more likely to remain within the organization as bedside nurses.

# CONCLUSION

Well, that's our story. We set out to create an innovative model focused on empowerment and engagement to create a career at the bedside and ultimately improve nurse retention. It wasn't easy, but we did it.

In truth, the program amounted to much more than we could have imagined. We had no idea that the program we built would affect as many people—indeed, the organization as a whole—as it has. Thanks to continued buy-in among organizational leaders and nurses alike, the program remains successful today.

If you read this book, you're probably looking for similarly positive outcomes in the areas of empowerment, engagement, and retention. To achieve that, start by asking yourself these questions:

- Are we empowering those who are closest to the work to make the difference we need to thrive in the future?

- Are we leading—rather than simply managing—our clinical nursing staff?

- Do we partner with our clinical nursing staff and allow them to lead with us?

If you could not answer "yes" to each of these questions, it is time to rethink your strategy.

Now ask:

- What if you had a program that fostered a culture that helped you meet your organization's strategic initiatives, mission, and vision?

- What if you had a program that ignited professional growth among nurses and promoted their retention?

- What if you had a program that positively affected patients and improved outcomes across the continuum of care?

As organizational leaders, we should always be looking for long-term, sustainable programs that lead us into the future. This is vital. There are so many things outside our control that can pull staff in other directions—especially if they do not feel supported and fulfilled in their roles. This is why, even during the recent pandemic, the IMPACT Model remained a key focus and continued in full force—payouts and all.

It is time to think differently—to stop reacting, to stop applying quick fixes that don't address the root of the problem. It's time to embrace nurses who don't want to leave the bedside but who are craving so much more. They will guide your organization to new horizons . . . *if you let them.*

# *REFERENCES*

DiNapoli, J. M., O'Flaherty, D., Musil, C., Clavelle, J. T., & Fitzpatrick, J. J. (2016). The relationship of clinical nurses' perceptions of structural and psychological empowerment and engagement on their unit. *Journal of Nursing Administration, 46*(2), 95–100.

George, V., Burke, L. J., Rodgers, B., Duthie, N., Hoffmann, M. L., Koceja, V., Kramer, A., Maro, J., Minzlaff, P., Pelczynski, S., Schmidt, M., Westen, B., Zielke, J., Brukwitzki, G., & Gehring, L. L. (2002). Developing staff nurse shared leadership behavior in professional nursing practice. *Nursing Administration Quarterly, 26*(3), 44–59.

Maslow, A. H. (1943). A theory of human motivation. *Psychological Review, 50*(4), 370–396. https://doi.org/10.1037/h0054346

# Explanation of Activities

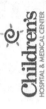

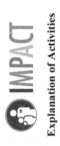

Children's
HOSPITAL & MEDICAL CENTER

**Explanation of Activities**

| Activity | Description of Clinical Activity (Level 1) | Submit |
|---|---|---|
| Evidence-Based Practice (EBP) Project | **Must be pre-approved (see EBP \| PI \| Research form)**<br><br>RN had an active role in EBP project using an EBP model (e.g., Johns Hopkins Nursing EBP Model, Iowa Model, etc.).<br><br>RN leads or co-leads an EBP project with a limited scope (e.g., impact on a single unit or narrow aspect of patient care on single unit).<br><br>**Must include the following points in your narrative (you may consider using these topics as headings):**<br><br>• Your role in EBP project<br>• Background to support project<br>• PICO question<br>• Collection and synthesis of evidence<br>• Description of how EBP project was implemented or communicated to specific area(s)<br>• EBP outcomes (or anticipated impact)<br>   o Recommendations for change and your involvement in the implementation of change<br>   o What measures are in place to monitor sustainment of outcomes?<br>   o If project ends in "no change" due to insufficient evidence or current practice is already evidence-based, please explain to receive activity points<br>• Lessons learned<br><br><br>**1 Project with Active Role = 1 Activity Point**<br><br>**1 Project Lead/Co-lead = 2 Activity Points** | ☐ **EBP \| PI \| Research form (Level 1)**<br><br>☐ **Literature Review table**<br><br>☐ **Benchmark table** (if appropriate)<br><br>☐ **PowerPoint report**<br><br>☐ **Education plan**<br><br>☐ **Any Policy/Procedures changed**<br><br>☐ **EBP Project Narrative:**<br>• Typed<br>• Double-spaced<br>• 12-point font |

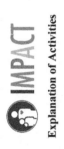

**IMPACT**

**Explanation of Activities**

**Children's**
HOSPITAL & MEDICAL CENTER

| Activity | Description of Clinical Activity (Level 2) | Submit |
|---|---|---|
| **Evidence-Based Practice (EBP) Project** | **Must be pre-approved (see EBP \| PI \| Research form)**<br><br>RN leads or co-leads an EBP project using an EBP model (e.g., Johns Hopkins Nursing EBP Model, Iowa Model, etc.) with an impact across multiple areas.<br><br>**Must include the following points in your narrative (you may consider using these topics as headings):**<br><br>• Background to support project<br>• PICO question<br>• Collection and synthesis of evidence<br>• Recommendations to multiple areas/committees<br>• Use of interprofessional team to translate recommendations into practice<br>• Your role in EBP project<br>• How you collaborated, facilitated, and coordinated project across all areas impacted<br>• Description of how EBP project was implemented or communicated to specific areas<br>• EBP outcomes (or anticipated impact)<br>• Implementation of change<br>• What measures are in place to monitor sustainment of outcomes/change?<br>   o Note: if project ends in "no change" due to insufficient evidence or current practice is already evidence-based, goes to a Level 1 submission<br>• Lessons learned<br><br><div align="center">**1 Project = 4 Activity Points**</div> | ☐ **EBP \| PI \| Research form (Level 2)**<br><br>☐ **Literature Review table**<br><br>☐ **Benchmark table (if appropriate)**<br><br>☐ **PowerPoint report**<br><br>☐ **Education plan**<br><br>☐ **Any Policy/Procedures changed**<br><br>☐ **EBP Project Narrative:**<br>  • Typed<br>  • Double-spaced<br>  • 12-point font |

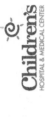

# IMPACT

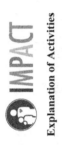

## Children's
### HOSPITAL & MEDICAL CENTER

## Explanation of Activities

| Activity | Description of Clinical Activity (Level I) | Submit |
|---|---|---|
| Performance/Quality Improvement Project | **Must be pre-approved (see EBP \| PI \| Research form)**<br><br>RN had an active role in a performance improvement initiative using a quality improvement model (e.g., PDCA, DMAIC, etc.) over and above unit-based expectations.<br><br>RN leads or co-leads a project with a limited scope (e.g., impact on a single unit or narrow aspect of patient care on single unit).<br><br>**Must include the following points in your narrative (you may consider using these topics as headings):**<br><br>• Description of process/quality improvement project<br>• What data was used to drive decisions<br>• Use of a quality improvement model (explain)<br>   ○ How you communicated/educated small tests of change for focused area/issue<br>• Who is affected by change (i.e., nursing only, interdisciplinary, etc.)<br>• How the change was implemented<br>• Your direct contributions to the project (skills/experience used)<br>• Material developed (i.e., PowerPoint, educational sheet, etc.)<br>• Outcomes of the project<br>   ○ Must show at least three post-data points<br>• Lessons learned<br><br>**1 Project with Active Role = 1 Activity Point**<br>**1 Project Lead/Co-lead = 2 Activity Points** | ☐ EBP \| PI \| Research form (Level I)<br><br>☐ Team Charter<br><br>☐ Other tools (workflow, fish bone, timelines, etc.)<br><br>☐ Report of outcomes in graph form<br><br>☐ Any Policy/Procedures changed<br><br>☐ PI Project Narrative:<br>   • Typed<br>   • Double-spaced<br>   • 12-point font |

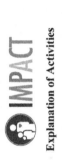

**IMPACT**

Children's
HOSPITAL & MEDICAL CENTER

## Explanation of Activities

| Activity | Description of Clinical Activity (Level II) | Submit |
|---|---|---|
| **Performance/Quality Improvement Project** | **Must be pre-approved (see EBP \| PI \| Research form)**<br><br>RN leads or co-leads a performance improvement initiative using a quality improvement model (e.g., PDCA, DMAIC, etc.) over and above unit-based expectations with impact across multiple areas.<br><br>**Must include the following points in your narrative (you may consider using these topics as headings):**<br><br>• Description of process/quality improvement project<br>• What data was used to drive decisions<br>• Use of a quality improvement model (explain)<br>   ○ How you communicated/educated small tests of change to multiple areas<br>   ○ System impact (minimum of two different types of areas such as clinic and inpatient nursing)<br>• Who is affected by change (i.e., nursing only, interdisciplinary, etc.)<br>• How the change was implemented<br>• Your direct contributions to the project (skills/experience used)<br>• Outcomes of the project (sustainment)<br>   ○ Must show at least three post-data points on at least two metrics/goals<br>• Lessons learned<br><br><div align="center">**1 Project = 4 Activity Points**</div> | ☐ **EBP \| PI \| Research form (Level II)**<br><br>☐ **Team Charter**<br><br>☐ **Other tools (workflow, fish bone, timelines, etc.)**<br><br>☐ **Report of outcomes in graph form**<br><br>☐ **PowerPoint report**<br><br>☐ **Education/communication developed**<br><br>☐ **PI Project Narrative:**<br>   • Typed<br>   • Double-spaced<br>   • 12-point font |

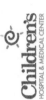

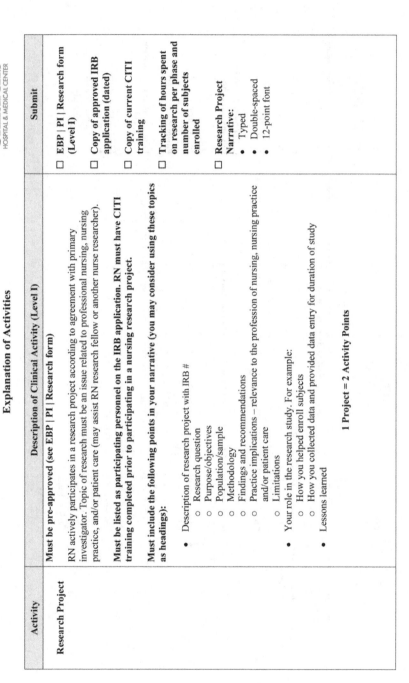

IMPACT

**Explanation of Activities**

Children's
HOSPITAL & MEDICAL CENTER

| Activity | Description of Clinical Activity (Level I) | Submit |
|---|---|---|
| Research Project | **Must be pre-approved (see EBP \| PI \| Research form)**<br><br>RN actively participates in a research project according to agreement with primary investigator. Topic of research must be an issue related to professional nursing, nursing practice, and/or patient care (may assist RN research fellow or another nurse researcher).<br><br>**Must be listed as participating personnel on the IRB application. RN must have CITI training completed prior to participating in a nursing research project.**<br><br>**Must include the following points in your narrative (you may consider using these topics as headings):**<br><br>• Description of research project with IRB #<br>  o Research question<br>  o Purpose/objectives<br>  o Population/sample<br>  o Methodology<br>  o Findings and recommendations<br>  o Practice implications – relevance to the profession of nursing, nursing practice and/or patient care<br>  o Limitations<br>• Your role in the research study. For example:<br>  o How you helped enroll subjects<br>  o How you collected data and provided data entry for duration of study<br>• Lessons learned<br><br>          **1 Project = 2 Activity Points** | ☐ **EBP \| PI \| Research form (Level I)**<br><br>☐ **Copy of approved IRB application (dated)**<br><br>☐ **Copy of current CITI training**<br><br>☐ **Tracking of hours spent on research per phase and number of subjects enrolled**<br><br>☐ **Research Project Narrative:**<br>• Typed<br>• Double-spaced<br>• 12-point font |

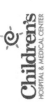

## Explanation of Activities

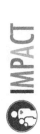

| Activity | Description of Clinical Activity (Level II) | Submit |
|---|---|---|
| **Research Project** | **Must be pre-approved (see EBP | PI | Research form)**<br><br>RN leads/co-leads a research project. Topic of research must be an issue related to professional nursing, clinical nursing practice, and/or patient care. RN must have CITI training completed prior to conducting or participating in a nursing research project (may co-lead with another RN research fellow or another nurse researcher).<br><br>**Must be listed as primary or secondary investigator on the IRB application.**<br><br>**Must include the following points in your narrative (you may consider using these topics as headings):**<br><br>• Description of research project with IRB #<br>   o Research question<br>   o Population/sample<br>   o Attach an electronic copy of the original research proposal & dated IRB application, and dated letter of approval<br>   o Include an electronic copy of abstract describing final research project including: introduction/literature review/gap, purpose/aims, methods, results, limitations, discussion, and practice implications<br>   o Describe (two to three sentences) contributions of the research project:<br>      ▪ Primary contribution/relevance to nursing practice, patient care, or addition to existing body of knowledge<br>• Describe (one paragraph) how you led and coordinated:<br>   o Overall development of the research project<br>   o Enrollment phase<br>   o Collection, management, and analysis of research data (include training of others in research processes)<br>   o Include the process of transparency/communication with stakeholders throughout all research phases<br>• Lessons learned<br><br>              **1 Project = 4 Activity Points** | ☐ **EBP | PI | Research form (Level II)**<br><br>☐ **Copy of approved IRB application (dated)**<br><br>☐ **Copy of IRB letter of approval (dated)**<br><br>☐ **Copy of current CITI training**<br><br>☐ **Research Project Narrative:**<br>   • Typed<br>   • Double-spaced<br>   • 12-point font |

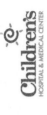

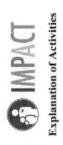

**Explanation of Activities**

| Activity | Description of Clinical Activity | Submit |
|---|---|---|
| **Clinical Special Project** | RN participates in a special project related to a clinical aspect of patient care. Multiple projects can be used to equal 4 hours.<br><br>• Some applicable activities include but are not limited to: Development of a new or innovative process related to direct patient care, patient safety, nurse sensitive indicators (healthcare-acquired conditions [CLABSI, CAUTI, falls]), etc.<br><br>**Must include the following points in your narrative (you may consider using these topics as headings):**<br><br>• Activity description<br>• Purpose/objectives<br>• Timeline (discuss when started and finished)<br>• What skill/experience you used for the project<br>• Material developed (i.e., PowerPoint, educational sheet)<br>• Outcomes of the activity<br>• Explanation of hours spent on project<br><br>**1 Activity = at least 4 hours** | ☐ **Activity Agreement form**<br><br>☐ **Supporting documents**<br><br>☐ **Narrative written for each project:**<br>• Typed<br>• Double-spaced<br>• 12-point font |

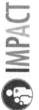
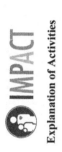

## IMPACT

### Explanation of Activities

**Children's**
HOSPITAL & MEDICAL CENTER

| Activity | Description of Clinical Activity | Submit |
|---|---|---|
| **Policy/Procedure Development or Change** | RN develops a new policy/procedure or updates an existing policy/procedure according to the most up-to-date evidence for best practice.<br><br>**Must include the following points in your narrative (you may consider using these topics as headings):**<br><br>• Description of process/quality improvement project<br>• How and why the change was implemented if revising policy<br>• Your contributions to the project<br>• How you met approval of CPC or under consideration (if house-wide policy and will affect more than your specific area); if you did not go through CPC, explain what approval process you went through<br>• Timeline (discuss when started and finished)<br>• What skill/experience you used for the project<br>• Material developed (i.e., PowerPoint, educational sheet)<br>• Outcomes of the activity<br>• Explanation of hours spent on project<br><br><div align="center">**1 Activity = 1 Policy/Procedure**</div> | ☐ **Activity Agreement form**<br><br>☐ **Copy of Policy (if new)**<br><br>☐ **Evidence-based research used to create or update the policy/procedure**<br><br>☐ **If policy/procedure updated, provide new and old policy to show changes**<br><br>☐ **Narrative:**<br>  • Typed<br>  • Double-spaced<br>  • 12-point font |

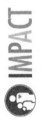
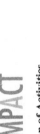

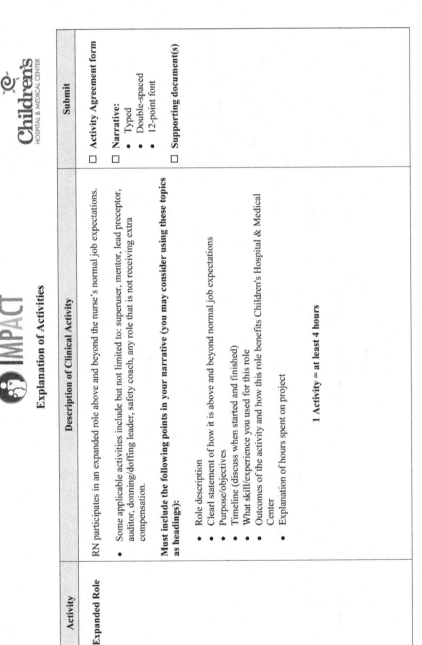

**Explanation of Activities**

| Activity | Description of Clinical Activity | Submit |
|---|---|---|
| **Expanded Role** | RN participates in an expanded role above and beyond the nurse's normal job expectations.<br><br>• Some applicable activities include but not limited to: superuser, mentor, lead preceptor, auditor, donning/doffing leader, safety coach, any role that is not receiving extra compensation.<br><br>**Must include the following points in your narrative (you may consider using these topics as headings):**<br><br>• Role description<br>• Clearl statement of how it is above and beyond normal job expectations<br>• Purpose/objectives<br>• Timeline (discuss when started and finished)<br>• What skill/experience you used for this role<br>• Outcomes of the activity and how this role benefits Children's Hospital & Medical Center<br>• Explanation of hours spent on project<br><br>**1 Activity = at least 4 hours** | ☐ **Activity Agreement form**<br><br>☐ **Narrative:**<br>• Typed<br>• Double-spaced<br>• 12-point font<br><br>☐ **Supporting document(s)** |

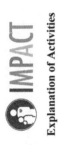

**Explanation of Activities**

## EDUCATION

| Activity | Description of Education Activity | Submit |
|---|---|---|
| **Contact Hours** **\*Required\*** (If you do not meet the minimum hours, the IMPACT portfolio will not be reviewed.) | Contact hours in continuing nursing education are a minimum requirement for Level I & II. Cannot include any mandatory hours (i.e., PALS, BLS, error prevention training, etc.) <u>Contact hour requirements:</u> **Level I = Minimum of 25** **Level II = Minimum of 31** | ☐ **Education form** ☐ **Copy of contact hour certificates (must have proof of hours)** |
| **Evidence-Based Inservice or Podium Presentation** | RN presents one evidence based inservice or poster presentation on an approved topic based on current evidence (does not include required report outs such as CORE PI projects). **Must include the following points in your narrative (you may consider using these topics as headings):** <ul><li>Goals/objectives of the poster/presentation</li><li>Who presented to?</li><li>Evidence used?</li><li>How it benefited the target audience</li><li>What you learned and/or what you would do different next time</li><li>Any potential next steps</li></ul> **1 Activity = 2 Different areas/departments presentations or 1 Hospital presentation** | ☐ **Presentation &** **Publications form** ☐ **Supporting document(s)** ☐ **Narrative:** <ul><li>Typed</li><li>Double-spaced</li><li>12-point font</li></ul> |

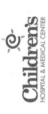

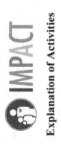

**Explanation of Activities**

| Activity | Description of Education Activity | Submit |
|---|---|---|
| **Instructor of Certification Course** | RN serves as an instructor for a certification course related to healthcare that is over and above job description expectations within 15 month time frame.<br><br>• Some applicable activities include, but not limited to: PALS, NRP, BLS, STABLE, etc.<br><br>**You must include the dates of the courses that you were the instructor.**<br><br>**1 Activity = 1 Course**<br>**Instructor for a minimum of 2 classes** | ☐ **Education form**<br><br>☐ **Copy of instructor card** |
| **Enrichment Course** | RN attends an enrichment course to enhance their knowledge within their current area of practice. Attendance is required; watching a recording of a course will not count. Contact hours may be offered but may not be used toward the contact hours required for IMPACT submission.<br><br>• Some applicable activities include but not limited to: organizational development courses, first year of EBP and research fellowship classes, presentations, grand rounds, etc.<br><br>**Must include separate narratives to explain how the courses are relevant to your nursing practice.**<br>• What has changed or been enhanced in your practice/knowledge of nursing after attending course(s)?<br>• What were your key learnings related to your current nursing practice as a direct patient nurse?<br><br>Multiple courses may add to equal 4 hours<br>**1 Activity = at least 4 hours** | ☐ **Activity Agreement form**<br><br>☐ **Supporting documents for each course** (certificate, cornerstone history, etc.)<br><br>☐ **Narrative for each course:**<br>• Typed<br>• Double-spaced<br>• 12-point font |

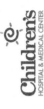

## IMPACT

### Explanation of Activities

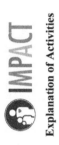

Children's
HOSPITAL & MEDICAL CENTER

| Activity | Description of Education Activity | Submit |
|---|---|---|
| **Healthcare Academic Courses** | RN successfully completes an academic course that leads to a degree in nursing and/or any academic course relevant to nursing practice taken for an academic credit. The RN must achieve a grade of "B" or higher or "pass" on a pass/fail system.<br><br>**Must include narrative to explain how the courses are relevant to nursing practice.**<br><br>• What has changed or been enhanced in your practice/knowledge of nursing after attending course(s)?<br>• What were your key learnings related to your current nursing practice as a direct patient nurse?<br><br>Multiple courses may add to equal 3 credit hours.<br><br>**1 Activity = 3 credit hours** | ☐ **Education form**<br><br>☐ **Copy of academic transcript**<br><br>☐ **Narrative for each course:**<br>  • Typed<br>  • Double-spaced<br>  • 12-point font |
| **Presentation within Children's Hospital & Medical Center** | RN presents and educates various staff within Children's Hospital & Medical Center (does not include required report outs such as CORE PI projects)<br><br>**Must include the following points in your narrative (you may consider using these topics as headings):**<br><br>• The goals/objectives of the presentation<br>  ○ Explain your specific role within the presentation<br>• How it benefited the target audience<br>• What you learned and/or what you would do different next time<br>• Any potential next steps<br><br>**1 Activity = 2 Department Presentations or 1 Hospital Presentation** | ☐ **Presentation & Publications form**<br><br>☐ **Narrative for each presentation:**<br>  • Typed<br>  • Double-spaced<br>  • 12-point font<br><br>☐ **Supporting document(s)** |

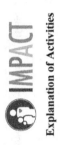

**IMPACT**

**Explanation of Activities**

**Children's**
HOSPITAL & MEDICAL CENTER

| Activity | Description of Education Activity | Submit |
|---|---|---|
| **Education Special Project** | RN participates or leads a special project related to an educational aspect of patient care or unit/hospital/system operations. Multiple projects can be used to equal 4 hours.<br><br>• Some applicable activities include but not limited to: family support project, support group, teaching skills, educating on EBP, etc.<br><br>**Must include the following points in your narrative (you may consider using these topics as headings):**<br><br>• Activity description<br>• Purpose/objectives<br>• Timeline (discuss when started and finished)<br>• What skill/experience you used for the project<br>• Material developed (PowerPoint, educational sheet)<br>• Outcomes of the activity<br>• Explanation of hours spent on project<br><br>**1 Activity = at least 4 hours** | ☐ **Activity Agreement form**<br><br>☐ **Narrative for each project:**<br>　• Typed<br>　• Double-spaced<br>　• 12-point font<br><br>☐ **Supporting document(s)** |

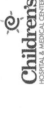

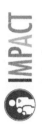

**Explanation of Activities**

## PROFESSIONAL

| Activity | Description of Professional Activity | Submit |
|---|---|---|
| **Specialty Certification *Required*** | RN has a specialty certification; must be in field of practice (i.e., PICU-CCRN, MS- CPN, etc.) within the 15-month submission time frame <br><br> **1 Certification = Required** | ☐ **Activity Agreement form** <br> ☐ **Copy of Certification** |
| **Additional Certification** | **Additional certification must include the following points in your narrative (you may consider using these topics as headings):** <br><br> • Description of additional certification <br> • How has the certification benefited you and Children's Hospital & Medical Center? <br><br> **1 Activity = Additional Certification** | ☐ **Activity Agreement form** <br> ☐ **Copy of Certification** <br><br> ☐ **Narrative for each certification:** <br>  • Typed <br>  • Double-spaced <br>  • 12-point font |
| Activity | Description of Professional Activity | Submit |

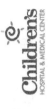

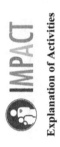

**Explanation of Activities**

| Committee/Council | Description of Professional Activity | Submit |
|---|---|---|
| | RN is/was an active member of a unit, hospital, or system committee or council for at least six months within the 15-month review period.<br><br>• Some applicable activities include but not limited to: shared governance council, CLABSI committee, developmental care committe, interdisciplinary committe, safety committee, P & T committee, etc.<br><br>**Must include the following points in your narrative (you may consider using these topics as headings):**<br><br>• Member for at least six months during the 15-month submission time<br>• Goals of committee/subcommittee<br>• Description of assignments you completed as an active member<br>• Description of what the committee has accomplished within the 15-month review period<br>• If you hold a co-chair position, description of your roles and responsibilities, including dates held (must hold co-chair position for at least six months)<br><br>1 Activity = Committee Member<br><br>2 Activities = Committee Co-Chair | ☐ **Committee/Subcommittee form**<br><br>☐ **Narrative for each committee/council:**<br>• Typed<br>• Double-spaced<br>• 12-point font |
| **Activity** | **Description of Professional Activity** | **Submit** |

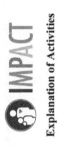

## IMPACT

## Children's
HOSPITAL & MEDICAL CENTER

### Explanation of Activities

| Activity | Description of Professional Activity | Submit |
|---|---|---|
| **Publication** | RN authors or contributes to publication.<br><br>**Must include the following points in your narrative (you may consider using these topics as headings):**<br><br>&bull; Description of what you contributed to the publication<br>&bull; The goals/objectives of the publication<br>&bull; How it benefited the target audience<br>&bull; What you learned and what would you do different next time<br>&bull; Any potential next steps<br><br>**2 Activities = National/Professional Level** | ☐ **Presentation & Publications form**<br><br>☐ **Narrative:**<br>&bull; Typed<br>&bull; Double-spaced<br>&bull; 12-point font<br><br>☐ **Copy of article and abstract** |

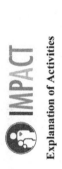

**IMPACT**

**Children's**
HOSPITAL & MEDICAL CENTER

**Explanation of Activities**

| Activity | Description of Professional Activity | Submit |
|---|---|---|
| **Presentation Outside of Children's Hospital & Medical Center** | RN presents poster or lecture at a city, state, regional, national, or international conference and/or program.<br><br>**Must include the following points in your narrative (you may consider using these topics as headings):**<br><br>• Location presented and audience presented to<br>• The goals/objectives of the presentation<br>• How it benefited the target audience<br>• What you learned and what you would do different next time<br>• Any potential next steps<br><br>**1 Activity = Local, State**<br><br>**2 Activities = Regional, National, or International Presentation** | ☐ **Presentation & Publications form**<br><br>☐ **Any handouts provided and/or picture of poster**<br><br>☐ **Narrative:**<br> • Typed<br> • Double-spaced<br> • 12-point font |

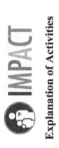

Children's
HOSPITAL & MEDICAL CENTER

IMPACT

## Explanation of Activities

| Activity | Description of Professional Activity | Submit |
|---|---|---|
| **Professional Organization Membership** | RN is an active member of a nursing professional organization for at least six months.<br><br>**Must include the following points in your narrative (you may consider using these topics as headings):**<br><br>• Member for at least six months during the 15-month submission time (must include year and/or months)<br>• Description of the meetings attended or the activities in which you are involved<br>• Why are you a member and how does it benefit you?<br>• If you hold an organization officer position, description of your roles and responsibilities, including dates of involvement and the contact information of a committee member<br><br>1 Activity = Membership<br><br>2 Activities = Organization Officer<br><br>(This activity can only be used one time) | ☐ **Professional Organization form**<br>☐ **Copy/verification of membership attached with year/months**<br><br>☐ **Narrative for each professional organization membership:**<br>• Typed<br>• Double-spaced<br>• 12-point font |

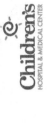

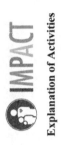

**Explanation of Activities**

| Activity | Description of Professional Activity | Submit |
|---|---|---|
| **Community Volunteer** | RN volunteers in the community in a non-health-related or health-related activity or in a leadership role and was not compensated for activity. Multiple volunteer activities can be used to reach the minimum of 6 hours.<br><br>**Must include the following points in your narrative (you may consider using these topics as headings):**<br><br>• Description of volunteer activity<br>• Purpose/objectives<br>• Timeline (discuss when started and finished)<br>• Skill/experience you used for the project<br>• Outcomes of the activity<br>• Explanation of hours spent on project<br><br>**1 Activity = at least 6 hours**<br><br>**(This activity can only be used one time and must be pre-approved prior to submission by a member of the IMPACT Committee.)** | ☐ **Activity Agreement form**<br><br>☐ **Narrative (per volunteer activity):**<br>    • Typed<br>    • Double-spaced<br>    • 12-point font |

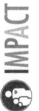
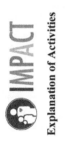

**IMPACT**

**Children's**
HOSPITAL & MEDICAL CENTER

**Explanation of Activities**

| Professional Special Project | RN participates in a special project related to professional aspects of patient care, professional practice, or unit/hospital/system operations. Multiple projects can be used to equal 4 hours. | ☐ Activity Agreement form<br>☐ Supporting document(s)<br>☐ Narrative (need separate for each project):<br>• Typed<br>• Double-spaced<br>• 12-point font |
|---|---|---|
| | • Some applicable activities include but not limited to: development of a new or innovative process that results in cost savings, time savings, or documented improved productivity, etc.<br><br>**Must include the following points in your narrative (you may consider using these topics as headings):**<br><br>• Project description<br>• Purpose/objectives<br>• Timeline (discuss when started and finished)<br>• What skill/experience you used for the project<br>• Material developed (PowerPoint, educational sheet)<br>• Outcomes of the activity (such as cost savings)<br>• Explanation of hours spent on project<br><br>**1 Activity = at least 4 hours** | |

## APPENDIX B

# Forms

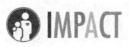 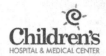

**Letter of Intent**

Name/Credentials:                   Employee ID #:

Department:       Years of Experience as an RN:         Current FTE:

Years in Current Specialty:       All Degree(s) Held:

Current Certifications:

Prior IMPACT Portfolio Submission       (Month/Year)

Level Submitting for: ☐ 1   ☐ 2

Intended Portfolio Submission Date:   ☐ April   ☐ October   Year:

I have reviewed and understand the IMPACT Education PowerPoint Presentation and Policy. ☐ Yes

RN Signature: _____     Date:

---

**Required Criteria**:
- Clinical, direct patient care registered nurse
- Works a minimum of 0.5 FTE (20 hours/week)
- Solid & Successful on annual evaluation/six month if new employee
- No active disciplinary action greater than a documented discussion in file

_____     _____
Manager/Supervisor Signature                Date

**Letter of Intent must be submitted at least four months prior to submission date:**
- Before June 1st for October submissions
- Before December 1st for April submissions

**Letter of intent**

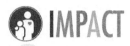 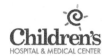

EBP | PI | Research Form Level 1

Applicant Name:

Clinical Activity: (Must have an Evidenced-Based Project, Performance/Quality Improvement Project, or Research Project)

| | |
|---|---|
| Evidenced-Based Project | ☐ |
| Performance Improvement | ☐ |
| Research Project | ☐ |

Project Title:

Project Dates:

Preapproved signatures required (prior to beginning project):

_____          _____
Clinical Educator/CNS                                    Clinical Manager

_____          _____
EBP | PI | Research Leadership                      Applicant RN Signature

_____
Validator Signature  (Must be the Project Leader or Mentor)
(As the validator you are attesting to the accuracy of the narrative written only, not the IMPACT Program requirements.)

**EBP, PI, & research activity form example**

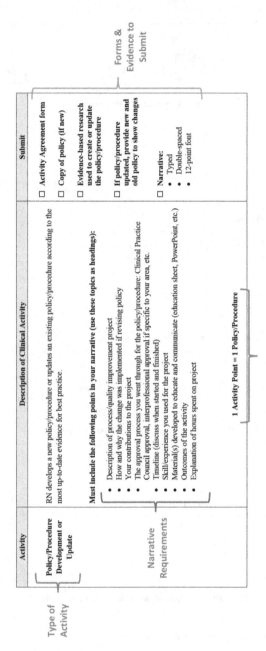

| Activity | Description of Clinical Activity | Submit |
|---|---|---|
| **Policy/Procedure Development or Update** | RN develops a new policy/procedure or updates an existing policy/procedure according to the most up-to-date evidence for best practice.<br><br>**Must include the following points in your narrative (use these topics as headings):**<br><br>• Description of process/quality improvement project<br>• How and why the change was implemented if revising policy<br>• Your contributions to the project<br>• The approval process you went through for the policy/procedure: Clinical Practice Council approval, interprofessional approval if specific to your area, etc.<br>• Timeline (discuss when started and finished)<br>• Skill/experience you used for the project<br>• Material(s) developed to educate and communicate (education sheet, PowerPoint, etc.)<br>• Outcomes of the activity<br>• Explanation of hours spent on project | ☐ **Activity Agreement form**<br><br>☐ **Copy of policy (if new)**<br><br>☐ **Evidence-based research used to create or update the policy/procedure**<br><br>☐ **If policy/procedure updated, provide new and old policy to show changes**<br><br>☐ **Narrative:**<br>  • Typed<br>  • Double-spaced<br>  • 12-point font |

**Type of Activity**

**Narrative Requirements**

**1 Activity Point = 1 Policy/Procedure**

**Activity Points Awarded**

**Forms & Evidence to Submit**

**Explanation of activities document example breakdown**

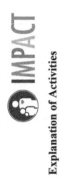

**IMPACT**

Children's
HOSPITAL & MEDICAL CENTER

## Explanation of Activities

| Activity | Description of Clinical Activity (Level 1) | Submit |
|---|---|---|
| **Evidence-Based Practice (EBP) Project** | **Must be preapproved (see EBP \| PI \| Research form)**<br><br>RN had an active role in an EBP project using an EBP model (e.g., Johns Hopkins Nursing EBP Model, Iowa Model, etc.).<br><br>RN leads or co-leads an EBP project with a limited scope (e.g., impact on a single unit or narrow aspect of patient care on single unit).<br><br>**Must include the following points in your narrative (use these topics as headings):**<br><br>• Your role in EBP project<br>• Background to support project<br>• PICO question<br>• Collection and synthesis of evidence<br>• How the EBP project was implemented or communicated to specific area(s)<br>• EBP outcomes (or anticipated impact)<br>   ○ What are your recommendations for change and your involvement in the implementation of change?<br>   ○ What measures are in place to monitor sustainment of outcomes?<br>   ○ If project ends in "no change" due to insufficient evidence or current practice is already evidence-based, please explain to receive activity points.<br>• Lessons learned<br><br>**1 Project with Active Role = 1 Activity Point**<br><br>**1 Project Lead/Co-lead = 2 Activity Points** | ☐ **EBP \| PI \| Research form (Level 1)**<br><br>☐ **Literature Review table**<br><br>☐ **Benchmark table (if appropriate)**<br><br>☐ **PowerPoint report**<br><br>☐ **Education plan**<br><br>☐ **Any policy/procedures changed**<br><br>☐ **EBP project narrative:**<br>   • Typed<br>   • Double-spaced<br>   • 12-point font |

Level 1 example for an EBP project requirements

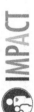

**IMPACT**

**Children's**
HOSPITAL & MEDICAL CENTER

## Explanation of Activities

| Activity | Description of Clinical Activity (Level 2) | Submit |
|---|---|---|
| **Evidence-Based Practice (EBP) Project** | **Must be pre-approved (see EBP | PI | Research form)**<br><br>RN leads or co-leads an EBP project using an EBP model (e.g., Johns Hopkins Nursing EBP Model, Iowa Model, etc.) with an impact across multiple areas.<br><br>**Must include the following points in your narrative (use these topics as headings):**<br><br>• Background to support project<br>• PICO question<br>• Collection and synthesis of evidence<br>• Recommendations to multiple areas/committees<br>• Use of interprofessional team to translate recommendations into practice<br>• Your role in EBP project<br>• How you collaborated, facilitated, and coordinated project across all areas impacted<br>• How EBP project was implemented or communicated to specific areas<br>• EBP outcomes (or anticipated impact)<br>• Implementation of change<br>• Measures in place to monitor sustainment of outcomes/change<br>  ○ Note: if project ends in "no change" due to insufficient evidence or current practice is already evidence-based, goes to a Level 1 submission<br>• Lessons learned<br><br>**1 Project = 4 Activity Points** | ☐ EBP | PI | Research form (Level 2)<br><br>☐ Literature Review table<br><br>☐ Benchmark table (if appropriate)<br><br>☐ PowerPoint report<br><br>☐ Education plan<br><br>☐ Any policy/procedures changed<br><br>☐ EBP project narrative:<br>  • Typed<br>  • Double-spaced<br>  • 12-point font |

**Level 2 example for an EBP project requirements**

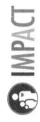 IMPACT

Explanation of Activities

Children's
HOSPITAL & MEDICAL CENTER

| Activity | Description of Professional Activity | Submit |
|---|---|---|
| **Presentation Outside of Children's Hospital & Medical Center** | RN presents poster or lecture at a city, state, regional, national, or international conference or program. <br><br> **Must include the following points in your narrative (use these topics as headings):** <br><br> • Location presented and audience presented to <br> • The goals/objectives of the presentation <br> • How it benefited the target audience <br> • What you learned and what you would do different the next time <br> • Any potential next steps <br><br> **1 Activity Point = Local or State Presentation** <br><br> **2 Activity Points = Regional, National, or International Presentation** | ☐ **Presentation & Publications form** <br><br> ☐ **Any handouts provided or picture of poster** <br><br> ☐ **Narrative:** <br> • Typed <br> • Double-spaced <br> • 12-point font |

**Example of how activity points are earned depending on the extent of work completed by the clinical nurse**

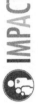

## IMPACT

### Explanation of Activities

**Children's** HOSPITAL & MEDICAL CENTER

| Activity | Description of Clinical Activity | Submit |
|---|---|---|
| **Expanded Role** | RN participates in an expanded role above and beyond the nurse's normal job expectations.<br><br>• Some applicable activities include, but not limited to: superuser, mentor, lead preceptor, auditor, donning/doffing leader, safety coach, and any role that is not receiving extra compensation.<br><br>**Must include the following points in your narrative (use these topics as headings):**<br><br>• Description of role<br>• How that role is above and beyond normal job expectations<br>• Purpose/objectives<br>• Timeline (discuss when started and finished)<br>• What skill/experience you used for this role<br>• Outcomes of the activity and how this role benefits Children's Hospital & Medical Center<br>• Explanation of hours spent on project<br><br><div align="center">**1 Activity Point = 4 hours minimum**</div> | ☐ **Activity Agreement form**<br><br>☐ **Narrative:**<br> • Typed<br> • Double-spaced<br> • 12-point font<br><br>☐ **Supporting document(s)** |

**Example of an activity in the clinical category**

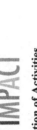

**IMPACT**

**Explanation of Activities**

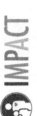

**Children's**
HOSPITAL & MEDICAL CENTER

| Activity | Description of Educational Activity | Submit |
|---|---|---|
| **Evidence-Based Inservice or Podium Presentation** | RN presents one evidence-based inservice or poster presentation based on current evidence. <br><br> **Must include the following points in your narrative (use these topics as headings):** <br><br> • The goals/objectives of the poster/presentation <br> • Who presented to <br> • Evidence used <br> • How it benefited the target audience <br> • What you learned and/or what you would do different next time <br> • Any potential next steps <br><br> **1 Activity Point = 2 Area/Department Presentations <br> or 1 Hospital Presentation** | ☐ **Presentation & Publications form** <br><br> ☐ **Supporting document(s)** <br><br> ☐ **Narrative:** <br> • Typed <br> • Double-spaced <br> • 12-point font |

Example of an activity in the educational category

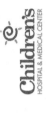

**Children's**
HOSPITAL & MEDICAL CENTER

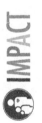

**Explanation of Activities**

| Activity | Description of Professional Activity | Submit |
|---|---|---|
| **Professional Organization Membership** | RN has been an active member of a nursing professional organization for at least six months. **Must include the following points in your narrative (use these topics as headings):** • Member for at least six months during the 15-month submission time (must include year and/or months). • Describe the meetings attended or the activities in which you are involved. • Why are you a member and how does it benefit you? • If you hold an organization officer position, please describe your roles and responsibilities, including dates of involvement and the contact information of a committee member. **1 Activity Point = Membership** **2 Activity Points = Organization Officer** (This activity can only be used one time.) | ☐ **Professional Organization form** ☐ **Copy/verification of membership attached with year/months** ☐ **Narrative for professional organization membership:** • Typed • Double-spaced • 12-point font |

**Example of an activity in the professional category**

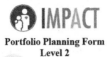

**Portfolio Planning Form**
**Level 2**

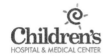

**Name/Credentials: Judy Thomas, BSN, RN, CCRN, CPN**

**Submission Date: 04/01/2021**

| | |
|---|---|
| **CLINICAL**<br>Must have an EBP, PI, or Research activity that impacts across the continuum of care<br>(Another area has been educated on the topic for potential/actual implementation) | ☑ |
| 1. **EBP Project: Nurse-Driven Foley Removal Algorithm** | |

| | |
|---|---|
| **EDUCATIONAL**<br>Four activities in at least three areas + at least 31 contact hours/year<br>(Must have an activity where you educated beyond your area a change in practice in which<br>you played a key role in dissemination of knowledge) | ☑ |
| Number of Contact Hours: **32.75** | |
| 1. **EBP Presentation: Nurse-Driven Foley Removal Algorithm to PICU Staff** | |
| 2. **EBP Presentation: Nurse-Driven Foley Removal Algorithm to Five Med-Surg Staff** | |
| 3. **Healthcare Academic Course: Nursing 722 Childcare Management** | |
| 4. **Enrichment Course: Pediatric Surgical Service Conference** | |

| | |
|---|---|
| **PROFESSIONAL**<br>Four activities in at least three areas + Specialty Certification<br>(Volunteer and professional organization membership can only be used once) | ☑ |
| Specialty Certification: **CPN** | |
| 1. **Additional Certification: CCRN** | |
| 2. **Committee Council: PICU HAC Committee** | |
| 3. **Professional Organization Membership: AACN** | |
| 4. **Community Volunteer: ENOA Meals on Wheels** | |

**Example of a completed level 2 portfolio planning form**

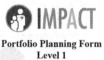 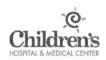

**Portfolio Planning Form**
**Level 1**

Applicant Name/Credentials: **Mellisa Renter, BSN, RN, CPN**

Submission Date: **04/01/2021**

| | |
|---|:---:|
| **CLINICAL**<br>Three activities in at least two areas<br>(Must have an EBP, PI, or Research activity) | ☑ |
| 1. **PI: Infusion Center FTE Utilization Improvement** | |
| 2. **Policy/Procedure Development: Rituxan** | |
| 3. **Expanded Role: Auditor CLABSI Standardization** | |
| **EDUCATIONAL**<br>Three activities in at least two areas + at least 25 contact hours/year<br>(Must have an evidence-based inservice or podium presentation) | ☑ |
| Number of Contact Hours: **25** | |
| 1. **Podium Presentation: Infusion Center FTE Utilization** | |
| 2. **Enrichment Course: Hunters Syndrome Presentation** | |
| 3. **Enrichment Course: Xatmep Medication Presentation** | |
| **PROFESSIONAL**<br>Three activities in at least two areas + Specialty Certification<br>(Volunteer and professional organization membership can only be used once) | ☑ |
| Specialty Certification: **CPN** | |
| 1. **Additional Certification: Chemotherapy and Biotherapy Provider** | |
| 2. **Professional Organization Membership: Association of Hematology Oncology Nurses – President** | |
| 3. **Professional Organization Membership: Association of Hematology Oncology Nurses – President** | |

**Example of a completed level 1 portfolio planning form**

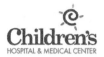

Judy Thomas, BSN, RN, CCRN, CPN

Thank you for your interest in the IMPACT Reward and Recognition Program at Children's Hospital & Medical Center. Your commitment to continue your clinical growth, professional development, and promotion of excellence in patient care is evident through the portfolio you submitted.

I am pleased to let you know that you have successfully met the initial requirements for the IMPACT Program Level 2 for April 2021. For the next step, please plan to present your portfolio information on **Tuesday, June 14th,** in the Glow Auditorium. Please arrive no later than 10:00 a.m.; the program will finish by 11:30 a.m. You will be receiving an email with the requirements regarding the presentation.

As the CNO/COO of Children's Hospital & Medical Center, I want to extend my gratitude for all you do and personally congratulate you on this remarkable achievement.

*Kathy English*

Kathy English, MSN, MBA, RN, FACHE
Executive Vice President,
Chief Nursing Officer, &
Chief Operations Officer

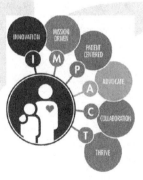

8200 Dodge Street | Omaha, NE 68114-4113 | 402-955-5400 | ChildrensOmaha.org

**Example congratulatory letter to advance to phase 3**

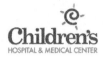

Mellisa Renter, BSN, RN, CPN

Thank for your interest in the IMPACT Reward and Recognition Program at Children's Hospital & Medical Center. Your commitment to continue your clinical growth, professional development, and promotion of excellence in patient care is evident through the portfolio you submitted.

I am pleased to let you know that you have successfully met the initial requirements for the IMPACT Program Level 1 for April 2021. For the next step, please plan to present your portfolio information on **Tuesday, June 14th**, in the Glow Auditorium. Please arrive no later than 10:00 a.m.; the program will finish by 11:30 a.m. You will be receiving an email with the requirements regarding the presentation.

As the CNO/COO of Children's Hospital & Medical Center, I want to extend my gratitude for all you do and personally congratulate you on this remarkable achievement.

*Kathy English*

Kathy English, MSN, MBA, RN, FACHE
Executive Vice President,
Chief Nursing Officer &
Chief Operations Officer

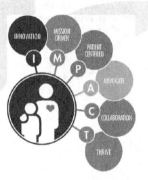

8200 Dodge Street | Omaha, NE 68114-4113 | 402-955-5400 | ChildrensOmaha.org

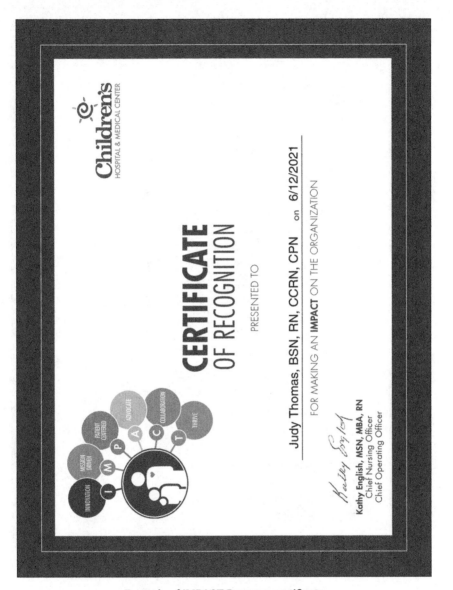

**Example of IMPACT Program certificate**

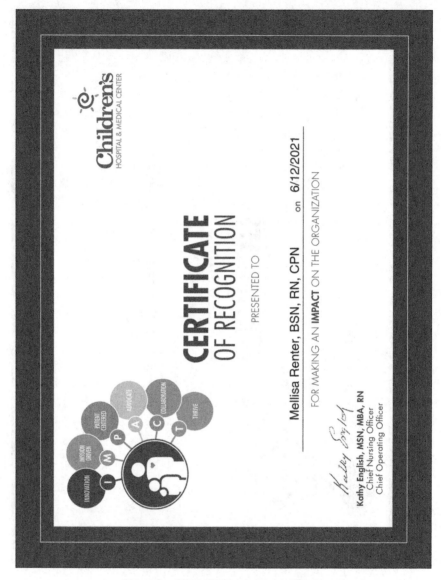

**Example of IMPACT Program certificate**

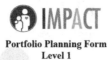
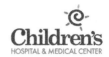

**Portfolio Planning Form**
**Level 1**

Applicant Name/Credentials: **Mellisa Renter, BSN, RN, CPN**

Submission Date: **04/01/2021**

| | |
|---|:---:|
| **CLINICAL**<br>Three activities in at least two areas<br>(Must have an EBP, PI, or Research activity) | ☑ |
| 1. **PI: Infusion Center FTE Utilization Improvement** | ☑ |
| 2. **Policy/Procedure Development: Rituxan** | ☑ |
| 3. **Expanded Role: Auditor CLABSI Standardization** | ☑ |
| **EDUCATIONAL**<br>Three activities in at least two areas + at least 25 contact hours/year<br>(Must have an evidence-based inservice or podium presentation) | ☑ |
| Number of Contact Hours: **25** | ☑ |
| 1. **Podium Presentation: Infusion Center FTE Utilization** | ☑ |
| 2. **Enrichment Course: Hunters Syndrome Presentation** | ☑ |
| 3. **Enrichment Course: Xatemp Presentation** | ☑ |
| **PROFESSIONAL**<br>Three activities in at least two areas + Specialty Certification<br>(Volunteer and professional organization membership can only be used once) | ☑ |
| Specialty Certification: **CPN** | ☑ |
| 1. **Additional Certification: Chemotherapy and Biotherapy Provider** | ☑ |
| 2. **Professional Organization Membership: Association of Hematology Oncology Nurses – President** | ☑ |
| 3. **Professional Organization Membership: Association of Hematology Oncology Nurses – President** | ☑ |

**Portfolio planning form: Level 1**

IMPACT

Portfolio Planning Form
Level 2

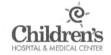

**Name/Credentials: Judy Thomas, BSN, RN, CCRN, CPN**

**Submission Date: 04/01/2021**

| | |
|---|:---:|
| **CLINICAL**<br>Must have an EBP, PI, or Research activity that impacts across the continuum of care<br>(Another area has been educated on the topic for potential/actual implementation) | ☑ |
| 1. <u>**EBP Project: Nurse-Driven Foley Removal Algorithm**</u> | ☑ |
| **EDUCATIONAL**<br>Four activities in at least three areas + at least 31 contact hours/year<br>(Must have an activity where you educated beyond your area a change in practice in which<br>you played a key role in dissemination of knowledge) | ☑ |
| Number of Contact Hours: **32.75** | ☑ |
| 1. <u>**EBP Presentation: Nurse-Driven Foley Removal Algorithm to**</u><br><u>**PICU Staff**</u> | ☑ |
| 2. <u>**EBP Presentation: Nurse-Driven Foley Removal Algorithm to**</u><br><u>**Five Med-Surg Staff**</u> | ☑ |
| 3. <u>**Healthcare Academic Course: Nursing 722 Childcare**</u><br><u>**Management**</u> | ☑ |
| 4. <u>**Enrichment Course: Pediatric Surgical Service Conference**</u> | ☑ |
| **PROFESSIONAL**<br>Four activities in at least three areas + Specialty Certification<br>(Volunteer and professional organization membership can only be used once) | ☑ |
| Specialty Certification: **CPN** | ☑ |
| 1. <u>**Additional Certification: CCRN**</u> | ☑ |
| 2. <u>**Committee Council: PICU HAC Committee**</u> | ☑ |
| 3. <u>**Professional Organization Membership: AACN**</u> | ☑ |
| 4. <u>**Community Volunteer: ENOA Meals on Wheels**</u> | ☑ |

**Portfolio planning form: Level 2**

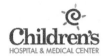

**Children's**
HOSPITAL & MEDICAL CENTER

[NAME],

Thank you for your interest in the IMPACT Reward and Recognition Program at Children's Hospital & Medical Center. During the review of your portfolio, there were key items missing, which prevents you from moving on to the presentation phase of the program.

We encourage you to continue working on your portfolio and activities for future submissions. Please contact Mellisa Renter, Director of Professional Nursing Practice, by email (mrenter@childrensomaha.org) or by phone (402-955-4180) if you would like to schedule a time to review your portfolio for future submissions.

Sincerely,

The IMPACT Review Committee

**Items Missing:**

- Level 2 Performance Improvement Project
  - o Outcomes of the project to prove sustainment
    - ▪ Must show three post-data points on at least two metrics/goals
  - o Team Charter

- Presentation within CHMC
  - o No supporting evidence submitted

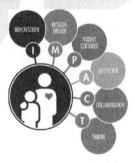

8200 Dodge Street | Omaha, NE 68114-4113 | 402-955-5400 | ChildrensOmaha.org

**Participant letter—missing components**

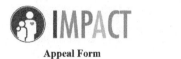 

**Appeal Form**

RN Name: _____    Date: _____

**IMPACT Appeal Process:**

- The applicant has 14 days to complete an appeal form and submit it to the Director – Professional Nursing Practice.
- Upon receipt of appeal request, the IMPACT Committee will schedule a meeting to review the applicant's portfolio and appeal.
- The appeal meeting will include at least two members of the IMPACT Committee, including a representative from Human Resources.
- The applicant will have 15 minutes to present their case to the IMPACT Committee.
- The IMPACT Committee will review the appeal and either approve or deny the appeal.
- The outcome will be forwarded in writing to the applicant within one week.

**Describe the reason for an appeal below:**

_____

_____

_____

_____

_____

**Applicant Signature:** _____

---

**Date Received by IMPACT Committee:** ____/____/____

**Interview Time/Date:** ____:____; ____/____/____

**Disposition of Appeal:** Approve _____ Reject _____ Date ____/____/____

**Comments:**

_____

_____

_____

**IMPACT Committee Signature:** _____    Date: _____

**IMPACT appeal form**

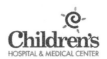

# IMPACT Recognition & Reward System
## April 2021 Presentations
## July 1, 2021 | 10:00 AM – 11:30 AM
## Glow Auditorium | Zoom

### AGENDA

**10:00 AM – 10:15 AM**
**Welcome and Introduction**

Mellisa Renter, MSN, RN, CPN
Director Professional Nursing Practice/MPD

Judy Thomas, MSN, RN, NEA-BC
Service Line Director H/O & Infusion Center

**10:15 AM – 11:00 AM**
**Presentations**

Kristen Foster, BSN, RN, CCRN (Transport RN)
*Evidence-Based Practice Project:*
*Using Manometers for ETT Cuff Pressure Measuring*

Lindsey Mittelbrun, BSN, RN, RNC-NIC (NICU RN)
*Performance Improvement Project:*
*CHG Hand Scrubbing in the NICU*

**11:00 AM – 11:30 AM**
**Award Ceremony & Final Remarks**

Kathy English, MSN, MBA, RN
Executive Vice President, CNO, COO

Mellisa Renter, MSN, RN, CPN
Director Professional Nursing Practice/MPD

Judy Thomas, MSN, RN, NEA-BC
Service Line Director H/O & Infusion Center

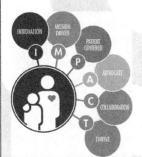

8200 Dodge Street | Omaha, NE 68114-4113 | 402-955-5400 | ChildrensOmaha.org

**Impact ceremony agenda**

# INDEX

NOTE: Page references noted with an *f* are figures.

# P–Q